The Fix is full of common sense and empowering information that is easily accessible for everyone. Whether or not you already have good health habits, this book is a must-read!

Dr. Jennifer Ju, M.D.
Family Practice Physician
Milford, Connecticut

Paddling successfully through the swamp of competing and self-defensive, self-justifying opinions, Dr Caldwell-Andrews provides an easy to follow road map to knowing the difference between what matters in health and what is just "sounding brass and tinkling cymbal."

The muck and quicksand of scientific fact is usually only half-represented so that a particular author can defend a particular bias. Adding to that the cross-whips of "big words" and "fancy science," authors' sequences often make their writing more complicated than a plate of sticky spaghetti —-resulting in sizzle but not steak when it comes to the confusing arena of "What actually and really does make a difference to my long-term health?"

Thank YOU, Dr. Caldwell-Andrews for a guide for the lay person that makes more difference than noise...and that will actually HELP folks live longer with "the right stuff"!

Dr. Russell L. Osmond
Change Strategies, International
Atlanta, Georgia

THE FIX

How a more integrative body-mind

approach creates lasting health

Alison Caldwell-Andrews**, PhD**

Cover Design: Kendall Bird
Illustrations and Artwork: Kendall Bird

Alison Caldwell-Andrews, PhD
www.mindbodytotalhealth.com
dr.alison@caldwellandrews.com

Dr. Caldwell-Andrews is not responsible for websites (or
their content) that are not owned by her.

ISBN-13:
978-1493594641

ISBN-10:
1493594648

To My Husband,
Who Forever Inspires Me

NOTE TO THE READER:

The information presented here is educational in nature, and represents the author's experience and opinion. This book is not intended as a substitute for medical advice from a physician. This book is intended as an information guide. The guidelines, techniques and approaches described in this book are not intended to treat, cure, prevent or diagnose any disease or to be a substitute for professional medical care, diagnosis or treatment. The author is not a medical doctor. You should consult with your physician before beginning any dietary, supplement or exercise regimen. A physician should be consulted if you are on medication or have any symptoms or concerns that may require diagnosis or medical attention. The data this book is based on may change in the future and, as a result, some of the conclusions drawn herein may become invalid as scientific advances continue. You should seek the most up-to-date information on your medical care and treatment from your physician or qualified health care professional. This book is not intended to treat or diagnose any condition that requires the services of a physician. This book is intended for educational purposes only.

THE FIX

Contents

Foreword

To me, the most interesting books are those that teach you something you didn't know, and do it in a way you enjoy. And, if they can cause you to look further into the subject and find even greater personal benefit or excitement (or at times even discomfort), they become something more. They become more than just a good read, or a fresh perspective. They become, to me, *a work*.

The Fix is just such a book, because it treats natural health in a way that either hasn't been articulated or hasn't been fully understood in the past. And it is clear that this book is just the beginning of much more to come — this is just the tip of the iceberg. For me, the personal benefits of reading it were evident from the first chapter.

My own strong feelings about mind and body natural health stem from very personal experiences in my own life and in the lives of people I am very close to, as well as from my 23 years of professional-life experiences. How my own feelings became impassioned enough to instill a sense of cause within me is not that much of a mystery, since my professional life allowed me to make hundreds upon hundreds of personal visits to homes, clinics and shops across the U.S.A. over many years. The sum of these involvements has left no doubt in my mind that everyone who lives on this planet is better off—

much better off—with herbs as a resource for daily health, including during life's toughest health challenges.

The existence, within this societal community, of both the desire for preservation of old ways and the desire for additional information and study has always been attractive to me, though that might run counter to some of the propaganda published about those who are open to natural solutions. Indeed, during all my years among this community I have witnessed an insatiable desire for any information regarding health, regardless of the specific health approach used, be it herbal, natural or otherwise integrated. One area where I have seen increased activity and study is that of the mind-body connection of various herbs and natural products.

It was during the time of my realization of this nascent evolution of the area of mind/body integrated natural health that I connected with Dr. Caldwell-Andrews. And since that time, I have been anticipating the release of her book. Whether you are new to the world of natural healing, or have decades of experience, this book will change the way you look at personal wellness. It will enhance your understanding no matter where you stand in terms of your practical use of herbal supplements or other natural products. And even if you don't yet see the worth of the nutritional side of mind-body health, there is much more contained in *The Fix* which I suspect you will find convincing enough to change the way you live for the better.

And that is really what I personally hope

the reader takes from this book, and why I have made mind/body integrated natural health my profession, as well. Thank you Alison, for helping us all move forward.

Greg Halliday
CEO Solle Naturals
Pleasant Grove, Utah
October 2013

Chapter One

Science and Synergy

veryone starts out in life with ideas about how the world works. Our brains do this for us automatically. Even infants can tell when a cup is close enough to the edge of a table so as to be in danger of falling off. Finding patterns in what we observe and identifying relationships between variables is a way of being human. It's part of being alive. We explain our world. We ascertain causality. We learn to predict.

And we think we are right.

Often we cling to ideas because they represent familiarity and safety. Sometimes it's useful to cling to past ideas. Sometimes it's impossible to let go. Sometimes letting go is fraught with anxiety, somewhat like jumping off a cliff. These experiences are all part of the human experience. Most of us have had moments when we figuratively did "jump off a cliff" in our search for truth, and found that there was no void after all.

The truth had been there all along.

We are all scientists in one sense or another. We all evaluate our observations about the world. In order to profit from our observations, we must be prepared to change what we believe is true when we find new information. We must constantly reevaluate in the light of our current experience.

Imagine you are learning to cook, and you believe that boiling everything is the right way to cook. If you are not able to question your assumptions about the importance of boiling, you'll never be able to truly taste the reality of what you've prepared! Your bias will make it so that you can't be a good observer. Boiling may stay "true" for you, but here's the outcome: you'll never be a great cook.

Science is the continual challenging of barriers to knowledge through acts of rigorous observation. Observation in this sense does not refer simply to scientific study design, research methodology and data collection, but to something more fundamental: It refers to our willingness to develop an awareness of how our biases affect the ways we perceive the world.

I'm referring to rigorously observing in the present moment so we can actually see what there is to be seen.

Nonetheless, we are limited. We don't know what we don't know. We cannot include variables that we don't understand. We may have glasses on our faces that we are unaware we are wearing!

One of the assumptions many of us cling to is the idea that we are more advanced, smarter and more sophisticated than people in previous eras were. Many of us still cling to the notion that the average person in Columbus' day truly believed the world was flat. We certainly believe that past eras were vastly inferior when it comes to health care. Indeed, modern-day advances are miraculous and some have the potential to be more life-saving than the medicine of ages past. But the existence of these advances doesn't mean that what we knew centuries ago was merely superstition. It also doesn't mean that modern medicine is always better, or is never harmful. For example, according to some experts, one of the leading causes of death in the United States is preventable harm resulting from medical treatment, or faulty advice to patients.

I find it interesting that in past eras, people in general used to find herbs much more useful, valuable and effective than we, as a people, find them today. I think the reason we don't see their effects as reliably in our modern times is that we have significantly changed the context we live in, and overwhelmed our bodies and minds. We are so laden with "baggage" that the herbal supports that used to help our ancestors don't seem to affect us the same way. Many herbs are mild enough to only provide a gentle nudge. Others are stronger. Then, there are some that are quite strong, so strong that they are rarely administered because they are dangerous. These last kinds of herbs are the ones that were grasped by the pharmaceutical industry and turned into medications. And they come trailing side effects.

Snake Oil and Salesmen

Certainly some of the prevailing herbal folklore of ages ago was superstition, and we can and should classify it as snake oil. Some of what is on the herbal and pharmaceutical markets today is also snake oil.

There always has been and there always will be snake oil and snake oil salesmen.

But it's a challenge to resist snake oil when you have no way of knowing what qualifies as snake oil. You may not know how to tell whether or not you're talking to a snake oil salesman. And sometimes the rock bottom fact is that the salesman doesn't even know that he or she is selling snake oil!

One of the more memorable experiences I had in graduate school was that of taking the required Qualifying Exams, covering everything we should have learned up to the end of graduate school. The Research Design and Methodology exam was one of my favorites. Since I am a total research nerd, this test examined my fun stuff: research methods and logic puzzles! I began it with enthusiasm. The object was to dismantle a published article and find any and all methodological and statistical errors. The more I looked, the more errors I saw. Some of them were glaring! I wondered where the article had been published, as that information had been blacked out in our copies. My first thought was to assume it must have been published in a very low-quality journal. But as I continued to write my criticisms, I changed my mind about that. Sure enough, when I checked with the instructor after the exam, the article in question was from one of the top three journals in its area, a journal with a rejection rate of 90%! If 90% of the articles submitted to this journal were rejected, you would think that the final 10% would be the cream of the crop. Not so. The article I had critiqued was an embarrassing methodological mess. I'll always remember the lesson I learned from that exam: just because you hear or read something from a respectable authority doesn't mean it's correct or even worthwhile.

Here's something to be aware of as you begin reading this book. If you haven't been accustomed to actively questioning "authority" or many of your own assumptions about health and common medical practices, you may find the first couple chapters of this book uncomfortable. In these early chapters, I raise many questions about conventional medical science as well as alternative modalities. It's fine for you to find these questions anxiety-provoking, annoying or dangerous. If you want to skip to later chapters for their practical information, feel free. You can always come back to the earlier chapters when you want more details about what makes science "tick."

Synergy is Primary

The concept of synergy underlies everything I write about in this book. Having good health is not merely about identifying a single problem or finding a single solution. Health is about synergy: the interactions between two or more variables, which result in effects that are either bigger than or different from the additive value of each of the individual variables.

Our modern scientific methods are not well designed to examine synergy. We are pretty good with problems that have single or even a few variables. We much prefer to examine one variable at a time in order to be certain of our results. So the idea of including synergy in studies rarely occurs to most of the folks who are running the lab coat shows. Synergy doesn't lend itself to a well-designed research study.

But the problem is that life doesn't happen at the speed of one variable at a time. Health is a context that includes everything in our lives and the manner in which all of those things affect each other. It may be that synergy has more to do with your health than any one particular health principle.

I observed a problem recently in a study that examined antioxidants in food. The author discussed what happened when the researchers extracted the antioxidants from food, put them into pills and administered them to humans. The researchers were surprised that the antioxidants didn't work as well as they had expected, based on how well those antioxidants had previously worked in the lab. So the study author concluded that, instead of antioxidants, there must be some other thing in the food that created its good effects.

What if it's the synergy created by foods—real, whole foods — that's good for us?! What if we can't ever reduce this synergy to a list of active ingredients because what's going on is ten-thousand variables' worth of synergy? What if the way we eat and digest food interacts with the way we prepare our food, as well as with the way our bodies have been interacting in the world for the past day, week, month and decade? What if all of those variables, plus the way the food was grown, harvested and marketed, affected our health outcomes? Happily, I see that some researchers are indeed coming to such conclusions. Synergy is an essential part of holistic thinking. Context is everything. Here's an example: You feel like you're coming down with a cold. You reach for help from the herb Echinacea. But, perhaps Echinacea is not going to work for you this time, not against the context of the rest of your life. You see, the use of Echinacea can be very complicated. Spring harvesting yields five times more of some of the beneficial ingredients as compared to fall harvesting. The root and leaf have different effects. If you start to take Echinacea the very moment you begin to feel sick, this early treatment makes a difference. If you're eating the Standard American Diet (SAD) that includes a high percentage of processed foods and antibiotic-laden meats, that SAD context may overwhelm the power of Echinacea.

So if a study attempting to determine the usefulness of Echinacea is carried out on people who carry a large burden of effects from the contexts they live in (i.e., diet, pollution, stress, etc.), that study may not show any positive effect of Echinacea. Lack of results here might mean more about context than about the value of that particular herb.

Finding Clarity

It takes a lot of formal education to become the kind of scientist who regularly publishes articles in medical journals. All of that schooling and experience compounded with scientists' personal history, result in many layers of bias upon bias, steeped in yet more bias. It's makes it hard to see anything with fresh eyes, and even harder if seeing with those fresh eyes threatens scientific ego. Sometimes experts are so full of hubris that they are blind.

When we are attached to being right, or when we become panicked about feeling unsafe because the world just offered us a startling new idea that doesn't fit into our beliefs, we are much less able to have moments of clarity.

But real breakthroughs are made by those who can live with that panic, and still step over their conventional lines in the sand.

Real learning happens when we begin, with our experienced eyes, to practice seeing through the eyes of a beginner. Thus instead of simply hearing "sound and fury," we begin to hear music.

The poet, Rilke said it well:

> *"I tell you that I have a long way to go before I am—where one begins....*
> *You are so young, so before all beginning, and I want to beg you, as much as I can, to be patient toward all that is unsolved in your heart and to try to love the questions themselves like locked rooms and like books that are written in a very foreign tongue. Do not now seek the answers, which cannot be given you because you would not be able to live them. And the point is, to live everything. Live*

*the questions now. Perhaps you will
then gradually, without noticing it,
live along some distant day into the
answer.*

*Resolve to be always beginning—to
be a beginner!"[1]*

There are principles in this book that I
currently think are correct. But I could be wrong.
They are based on the best knowledge that I
possess right now, and empirical knowledge is
always subject to change.

In fact, just today I saw an article that ran
counter to something I'd thought was correct for
many years. It was research showing that being
angry actually lowers cortisol instead of raising it.
Based on past research about this subject, what I
had previously "known" was that our feeling any
threat, including being angry, raised cortisol
levels.

I had to re-evaluate my thinking. Apparently our bodily response to strong emotions is
even more complicated than I had known. I
didn't like my experience of reading that
research. It made me question a "truth" I thought
I knew. I wanted to walk away. I wanted to find
flaws in the study. But when I looked into the
research, it wouldn't cooperate with being wrong!
Instead I found a confirming study.

It was uncomfortable to find out that

---

[1] Translation by John Moody

something I'd been teaching people for years may no longer be true. I had a choice: if I just ignored the information, no change in my life would be necessary and my position could remain "right." At least for a few more years.

But being right is not the same thing as being effective.

I choose to be effective.

And I choose to have integrity. I can't ignore what I see without losing who I am.

So now I get to fit these new data about anger and cortisol into my understanding of how things work. This continual re-fitting into an ever changing world of understanding makes being human exciting!

To reiterate, true scientists keep learning and re-forming their opinions. Scientific rigor includes refusing to seek "ego" safety by clinging to static ideas about how the world works. Science is a commitment to constantly evaluate what you think you know, and compare it to what you are currently finding out. We identify what appears to be truth in the moment and we then temporarily rest on those ideas as we continue to figure out more about the world.

This book is not Guaranteed Truth. It's a journey toward the truth, a fun journey about You. And right now, what I share with you in this book is as close to my understanding of truth as I have been able to come to, thus far.

This is my current story about how health "works." This book is about tapping into the pervasive power of the mind-body connection. It's about context and about synergy. It's about behavior, including your thoughts, your emotions and your actions. It's about six Big Ideas that I hope will change your life.

My fondest hope is that you will use this book to help you in your journey of continually, honestly reevaluating what you know and what you daily do with the fundamental instrument of your life: your whole Self — mind and body.

Chapter Two

Mind -Body Connections

Y ou are reading this now because you have some interest in feeling good. Great start! I want to keep you encouraged and add even more motivation and information to help you in your quest to feel good.

People talk about feeling good as if it's a wonderful gift, and it is, but it's a gift we *all* can earn. It's not about luck or fate. We may have certain limitations, but within those limitations we all can learn what we need to do to feel good.

We are in a health crisis, certainly in the United States, but also in the world. Traditional health care is expensive and out of reach for many people. Medications may help sometimes but they don't always help and often not without unwanted side effects. Medication side effects have caused the largest popular backlash against conventional medicine in memory. More and more people are turning to alternatives — and there are a growing number of available options!

Much of conventional medicine lumps all the alternative options together (they are actually termed Complementary and Alternative Medicine, or CAM) and turns them into a giant mish-mash of hokey cures which are often considered entirely opposed to conventional medicine. Much of the public has the perception that all of these alternatives are equally hokey. When I walked the hallowed halls at the Yale University School of Medicine just a decade ago, that environment was filled with a strong sense of contempt and disregard for CAM in any form. Chiropractic, homeopathy, herbal, and even plain behavioral medicine were all met with varying degrees of sneer. I ran into bias when designing research, writing grants and publishing articles. Even though I had been hired specifically to work in the area of mind-body medicine, I was told I couldn't publish certain statements despite what the data were telling us, because they were "politically incorrect" or "no one will believe it," and my favorite: "We can't publish that – we are funded by [a pharmaceutical company] and this will make them unhappy." And these responses were applied to research in the area of behavioral medicine, an area that, compared to many other CAM approaches, enjoyed some status as a fairly legitimate and well-tolerated alternative to drugs.

Unfortunately I am not alone in this kind of experience.

Mind-body medicine is founded on the premise that the body and the mind are inseparably connected. This idea is ancient. It was a core understanding of healing practices in both traditional Chinese medicine and the Ayurvedic cultures. But according to our present-day conventional medical world's ideal of objectivity, separating the mind from the body has been seen as progressive and more scientific. After all, the thinking has been that you can measure things in the body objectively, but you cannot measure thoughts and feelings nearly as objectively.

> *Mind-body medicine is founded on the premise that the body and the mind are inseparably connected.*

The usefulness of objective measurement, however, also depends on knowing what all the relevant variables are, tracking them appropriately, and then identifying and understanding all potential causal factors. With recent advances in understanding particle physics, and inexplicable findings from ventures in vibrational science as just two examples, it is clear that we cannot pretend to know all the relevant variables and how they may affect one another.

Simply put, the scientific method works. But it only works within in the context of understanding the limits to what we may achieve. Many studies cannot identify all relevant variables, control what needs to be controlled or measure outcomes precisely enough to be truly objective. Our biases and lack of knowledge are possibly the most influential factors in controlling what we can rely on in scientific studies to date.

What is Mind-Body Medicine?

Mind-body medicine is not the same thing as Complementary and Alternative Medicine (CAM); however, they are linked. Many CAM treatments are firmly oriented in a mind-body understanding of health. In contrast, little of conventional medicine is based in the assumption that the mind and body are inextricable. Most physicians recognize that their patient's moods will affect recovery or disease prognosis, but mind-body medicine is far more than an acknowledgement that one's mood can affect one's physical functioning. Yet when we focus on our health, we often leave out the mind, unless you count motivational speeches, meditation, yoga, and good attitudes.

There is a vast amount of research that supports the mind-body connection and provides evidence for alternatives to conventional medicine that work within the mind-body context. This is what *The Fix* is about. I want to share with you some of these research gems. In reality, there's usually a substantial time gap between scientific discovery and the implementation of those discoveries. What this means is that even though a study may have been published, it typically takes over a decade (often close to two decades) before that research actually becomes part of medical practice. This book goes right to the scientific literature and pulls from some of the most salient and up-to-date research.

What we learn from that body of cutting-edge research is simply this: If you want to get better, you need to harness the powers of both your mind *and* your body.

To illustrate, if you want to be healthy, you can't just exercise and stay bitter at your ex. You can't work on forgiveness and then overeat four days a week. Sure, you may be informed enough to use some good quality supplements. But although using supplements can be an important part of addressing specific problems, they are not the route to vibrant health.

Another potential weakness of conventional medicine is that there's a tendency to separate into arbitrary parts what are usually very complex, integrated and interactive events. Think about this all-too-common scenario: You are diagnosed with allergies, then down the road you end up with Type II Diabetes and along the way you picked up some lower back pain. Whatever the condition is, there's a medication for it, so by the time you hit middle age you're on about six medications, plus maybe a couple to address the side effects of the first ones. It's kind of like, "There's an app for that," except it's "There's a medication for that.[b]" Your friends tell you that's just what happens when you get older, and since they are on nearly as much or more medication than you, it's very easy to fall into the trap of believing that this is just the way it is. It's hard to make sure that each of your doctors is keeping good track of all the medications you are on so that the new ones they prescribe don't interfere with what you're already on. What a mess!

---

[b] This fun analogy is from Dr. Mack Stephenson.

It seems clear that one of the problems with the current medical care system is that most medical doctors are not trained to think holistically – they are trained to be specialists. They choose an area to specialize in while they are still in school and that becomes their world. You remember the old saw, "When all you have is a hammer, everything looks like a nail." Doctors are trained to see illness in terms of how those symptoms relate to their area. Here's a personal example of a time when that saying played out in my medical care: Many years ago I went to three different doctors, hoping to find relief from a chronic cough. My cough received three different diagnoses. The general practitioner told me it was probably allergies. An ENT told me it was definitely reflux (GERD), and an internist said it was asthma. Each had their own particular hammer and my cough was just another nail. Worse, none of their treatments had any appreciable effect on the cough!

Another example highlights how inter-connected our problems are and how divided our treatment has become:

Most primary doctors will probably see severe asthma as two things:

1) A management problem (something the doctor has to keep track of over time), and

2) Something to refer out to a pulmonary specialist.

The pulmonary specialist will work to help resolve the asthma, but then will probably end up referring this patient to another specialist — a GI specialist — because, in connection to asthma and its treatment, the patient now has irritable bowel syndrome. Oh, and don't forget the extra dental work needed when those asthma medications wreak havoc in the mouth!

Many physicians are really quite good, and they may know a lot about their specialties, but far fewer are able to take the time to truly think about the person as a whole and to identify underlying causes as opposed to leaping to band-aid solutions. For example, asthma and irritable bowel syndrome may share an underlying cause (stress and its resulting chronic inflammation) but how many times do you think you'll be sent to a psychologist for help with asthma and IBS? After all, managed care doesn't really pay for identifying underlying causality when a band-aid fix is a "usual and customary" practice.

Primary care physicians have a hard time of it. Their patients are demanding. Their insurance reimbursements are being driven lower and lower. With office overhead, malpractice insurance costs, and student loans to repay, they actually can't financially afford to sit down with you for a long enough time to effectively individualize your treatment. It's not that they are trying to make you feel like a body in line, but a thirty or even twenty-minute appointment cuts significantly into their ability to cover all their expenses. Specialists have an easier time of it because they can demand higher levels of reimbursement, but the problem here is that they've been trained to see one thing. Specialists can be incredibly helpful but they are not generally in the business of looking outside of what they do for an alternative proximal cause of your problem. Like I said, when all you have is a hammer, everything starts to look like a nail.

The current medical system isn't working even close to its ideal, and it's important to recognize that it's not because physicians don't care, or because they are all out to get you. Many of those doctors are doing the best they can in a flawed system. But the problem is that *you* are caught up in that system, and you are the one with the fatigue, the cravings, the back pain, the weight gain, the insulin resistance, and the side effects – from both the medication and all that frustration or guilt.

One of the messages of this book is that there are some basic underlying causes to the many, many medical problems that most Americans face. When the body is treated as a combination of separate organ systems, it's hard to identify underlying causes. It's easy to get distracted with multiple problems to tackle, including a variety of physical problems, relationship problems, financial problems, spiritual problems, etc. — the full catastrophe. Our health suffers and we push through, thinking we'll find time for our health later. Or we try to take care of our health and our caretaking makes things worse because that caretaking is based on an inaccurate understanding of how body and mind are inextricably connected.

We don't think that any of you will argue that the system works just fine as it is.

The mind-body approach urges you to treat yourself as a whole being. For example, if you struggle with Type II Diabetes, it's far more effective to engage your whole self in that struggle as compared to merely popping some bitter melon extract and drinking some holy basil tea (both of which have good blood sugar effects, by the way).

Engaging the whole person means not thinking about mind vs. body but rather treating the body as mind and the mind as body. It's far more than engaging the mind as a form of motivation or source of positive attitudes. It's more than practicing some meditation. It's a whole different way of thinking. And that's the point – it's not a mere change in behavior or the popping of a different pill. It's a radical shifting of your worldview.

Holistic medicine is often misunderstood as the mumbo jumbo you get from quacks. Not so. Holistic medicine looks at everything you are – all the parts of your life that make up who you are – and treats you as a person with many dimensions (as opposed to, say, a gall bladder with a history). Conventional treatment can be a part of holistic medicine, as can chiropractic care or herbal medicine. To practice holistic medicine is simply to treat the person as a whole. This includes an understanding and appreciation of how the mind and body are one.

This book is not only about the psychological effects of particular disorders, or about how you can use your mind to overcome disease. It is more particularly about the inextricable connection between mind and body that exists and how this plays out in the way you take charge of your health.

You and I will take a look at a number of problems that many Americans struggle with, and we'll look at specific ways that body and mind work together to cause and to resolve these particular problems.

I'll focus a little bit on some non-pharmaceutical solutions, not because I have entirely abandoned the pharmaceutical industry but because there is plenty of information about those medications already on the market. What's needed is a description of alternative treatments that have empirical support. I want you to understand something of what science says about all that stuff you didn't learn much about in school. Let me be clear – I love the scientific method. I don't reject western science, in fact I embrace it despite its many flaws. What I hope to do is weave together an array of knowledge in ways that may surprise and inspire you. There's a lot of information out there that doesn't make it into the average medical school curriculum.

Let me give you more tools for your total health toolbox.

Chapter Three

One Thing Leads to Another

A young woman walked into my office, beautiful, capable, intelligent and chronically depressed. She had been depressed off and on (mostly on) since she was about 12 years old but managed to graduate from college, though it took her an extra year due to some hospitalizations. She currently had an excellent job. She had friends and a healthy social life. She had a family that she loved and felt loved by, she had a fantastic boyfriend, and she even played the clarinet in a local community orchestra. She had no history of trauma.

So why was she depressed?

We'll call her Maxine. I've changed some details to protect her identity, but you'll get the picture. As I talked to Maxine I found her to be very engaging, funny and candid. Her thinking was a little foggy, but aside from a tendency to be self-critical, her basic thought patterns were not problematic. She had no trouble falling asleep and staying asleep although she usually went to bed late. She was somewhat overweight and had tremendous trouble losing weight. She had very little energy. She said she sometimes had trouble getting out of bed and functioning, but not currently. She ate vegetables and tried to go to the gym, and when she managed to go, she pushed herself hard. She didn't smoke, drink excessively or do drugs. She admitted she had low self-esteem, and often treated herself harshly. And, as mentioned earlier, she was depressed.

Maxine had seen a dozen doctors who all said she was fine. They said her thyroid was fine, her blood sugar was fine, she didn't have a sleep disorder, and then they referred her to a psychiatrist for medication. She told me that in every case, as soon as the various specialists she consulted found out about her history of depression, each told her that her symptoms were because of her depression. That is a very common conclusion when no "medical cause" is found. Maxine described to me the discouraging repetitive scenario at each of her medical visits: how each of the specialists would be in the middle of gathering information, come to find out about her history of depression and then just stop instantly in their tracks. They would visibly quit pursuing other lines of concern as they would tell her that her symptoms were simply a result of depression.

I urged her to find a new physician in order to check things out more fully, because it seemed clear to me that her depression was primarily physiological.[c]

"It's not all in my head?" she asked, confused yet hopeful.

I shook my head. "No. Go find a doctor who doesn't tell you it's all in your head and who's willing to run more thorough tests."

And so she did. A more complete test of her thyroid functioning showed that although she had normal TSH (thyroid stimulating hormone) levels, her free T3 and T4 were low. Previous physicians had not seen these problems.

She also tested positive for Lyme disease. Both Lyme disease and hypothyroidism are known for their connection to depression.

As we discussed her history, including a long series of ear infections and antibiotic treatment as a child up to the gastrointestinal problems and irregular menses that plagued her now, her history of depression became more understandable and appeared more and more to be a physiological result of her overall health. What we saw was that throughout her as yet relatively short life, one thing had led to another, and here she was in my office, looking for change. Indeed, it was not "just in her head." Our focus soon became how to use her mind to help her body heal and how she could use her body to help heal her mind.

With this introduction, we now come to the first big idea of *The Fix:*

---

[c]We'll talk more about this idea in the chapter on depression.

Big Idea #1:
The Magic Bullet Paradigm:
As a society; we are stuck in the idea
that there is primarily one cause and
one cure for almost any ill.

What Magic Bullet Thinking Looks Like

You can see Magic Bullet thinking clearly in popular hospital-based television shows like *ER* or *Grey's Anatomy*. The storyline goes like this: problem, diagnosis, cure, all better. It plays out in the program like this: Patient comes in with mysterious symptoms. After trying multiple things with no luck (but plenty of drama), there is a triumphant diagnostic breakthrough! The right treatment is found, applied and the problem is fixed.

We replay this plot all the time to ourselves. "I feel awful. Why? It must be that soup I ate. No soup for me!" Of course we all want to identify the cause of what's wrong so we can fix it. Solving problems is a fundamentally human trait. But we are stuck thinking that there is one Magic Bullet solution to our ills and that if we can just find that one Magic Bullet, we will easily solve the problem. Problem – cause – Magic Bullet – cure.

Too much month at the end of your money? Problem: reckless spending, Magic bullet: budget. You're cured!

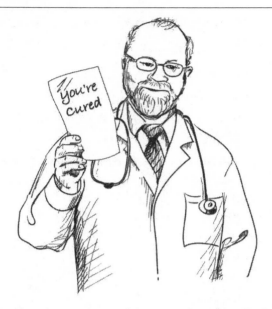

Germ theory? Problem: germs and therefore disease, Magic Bullet: get rid of the germs. You're cured!

Heart disease? Problem: high cholesterol, Magic Bullet: cholesterol lowering drugs/diet /lifestyle. You're cured!

Cancer? Problem: tumor, Magic Bullet: Take it out. You're cured!

So if there's one main cure for the one main problem, it's just a matter of finding the right fix. If you can't find that Magic Bullet, you either keep looking or you accept your fate. In Maxine's case, her doctors saw that she was depressed. Since there were no other findings indicating another problem, they assumed her symptoms were a result of depression — a reasonable assumption when you're seeing lack of energy, inability to lose weight, insomnia, discouragement and a history of depression. From the standpoint of conventional medicine, the problem was simply depression and therefore the treatment was to simply fix the depression.

We are all a bunch of caterpillars cocooned in familiar thinking.

The Strep Throat Example

Here's another example: Strep throat. I like to use this one because at first it seems so simple. I mean, we think we really *can* identify the one problem (group A streptococcus bacteria), one solution (antibiotics) and an outcome: strep throat is gone! A cure!.

If your throat is red and sore, you probably go to the doctor and get a strep test. If it's positive for strep, you get a prescription for antibiotics and take every last one. Or even if your doctor hesitates, you badger her into giving you antibiotics anyway despite the fact that 80% of sore throats are the result of viral infections and the antibiotic will do you no good. After all, one of the feared alternatives is rheumatic fever[d], followed by heart damage or death.

Here's reality, what the actual research says: Taking antibiotics does indeed shorten the duration of strep throat, but only by about 16 hours on average. Ibuprofen is cheaper, kinder to your body and will do a better job controlling the pain and inflammation. Whether you take antibiotics or not, strep throat is going to last between 3 and 5 days. More importantly, however, curtailing the strep throat symptoms

---

[d] Scarlet fever is another possible outcome occurring in about 10% of strep throat cases. If it occurs, it's easily treatable with antibiotics http://www.cdc.gov/features/scarletfever/

isn't really the point of the antibiotic. Although most people believe that they take antibiotics to treat the strep throat, the antibiotics are actually intended to prevent the possibility of rheumatic fever. Now don't get me wrong – I'm not advising you to NOT take the antibiotic, but encouraging you look at all the facts.

Looking at a broader picture, we realize that facts make this decision more complicated. The first complication is the fact that there are plenty of people who have that same strep bacteria[1] but none of the symptoms. They are just walking around and living normally, carrying strep bacteria. We don't know why this is. Physicians do not consider these "strep-carriers" to be an infection threat to others, nor do physicians believe that these people require treatment.[2] This fact doesn't fit into our neat little story very well, does it?

Next challenge to the prevailing wisdom: taking antibiotics won't entirely remove the risk of complications like rheumatic fever but rather merely *reduces* that risk. Sure, the reduced risk looks great on paper (the relative risk with antibiotics = 0.28[3] as compared to a "regular" risk of 1.0 in a case where risk has not been reduced at all) but here's the bigger picture: you have to factor in the reality that rheumatic fever is a very, very rare occurrence, even without antibiotics. In the early 1900's, before antibiotics, the incidence of rheumatic fever was about 5-10 cases per 1,000. Now it has dropped to less than 0.5 per thousand[4] by some reports, and fewer than 1 in a million by others[5]. Another source states that the incidence of rheumatic fever in the United States is so low that you'd have to give antibiotics to between 3,000 and 4,000 people in order to prevent just 1 case of rheumatic fever[6]. So although antibiotics do reduce the risk, that risk was pretty low to begin with. In fact, Dr. David Newman, MD, an expert on rheumatic fever, points out that since the rheumatic fever epidemic of the 1940s, the incidence of rheumatic fever has nearly disappeared in the United States[e] — so much so that the CDC has stopped tracking it. He also notes that because the nature of the pathogen changed, antibiotics probably were not the reason for the disappearance of rheumatic fever. Rather, improved hygiene and nutrition are more likely why we have nearly eradicated the disease in the United States (this also explains why rheumatic fever is still a problem in third-world countries today).

Still, your doctor will urge you to take antibiotics. Rheumatic fever isn't something you want to risk, so prevention is preferable.

But now there's more recent research that takes us around a whole new bend. It appears that susceptibility to rheumatic fever is less a matter of antibiotics, and instead appears to be largely genetic.[7] So it may be that who your parents are and what genes they bestowed on you are a better protection from rheumatic fever than antibiotics. Part of the reason for this is that rheumatic fever is not itself even caused by the same group A streptococcal bacteria that causes strep throat. That is, rheumatic fever is not directly caused by bacteria, but instead by a particular reaction within the body to that

---

[e] It was less than 1 case per million people.

bacteria. Rheumatic fever happens when the antibodies that were created by the immune system to fight off the streptococcal group A infection react with specific other proteins in the body. This genetically generated cross-reaction essentially causes the body to attack itself, resulting in what we call rheumatic fever.

Perhaps the rationale for antibiotic use is the thinking that if your body doesn't have to create antibodies in order to fight off the initial strep throat infection, then it won't have a chance to create antibodies that might cross-react, causing rheumatic fever. But your body creates antibodies right away — before you see your doctor for antibiotics.

In fact, it looks like antibiotics are no *guarantee* of safety from rheumatic fever after all. In a report detailing the rheumatic fever epidemic of the 1940's at Warren Air Force Base, Dr. Newman discussed statistics that showed when people were given antibiotics, less than 1% got rheumatic fever[8], indicating that some, albeit few, of the people who received antibiotics still got rheumatic fever. However, when people took a placebo rather than antibiotics, 2% got rheumatic fever. The points here are these: 1) antibiotics cannot guarantee that the risk of infection is 100% eliminated, and 2) the risk is low to begin with. And this was data from the 1940's during one of the worst epidemics of rheumatic fever we've known in this country. As stated previously, Dr. Newman pointed out that since the 1940's, the incidence of rheumatic fever has dropped dramatically due to better hygiene and nutrition. He followed up with this one-two punch idea: using antibiotics to prevent rheumatic fever these days makes about as much sense as administering antibiotics to the population in order to prevent a potential outbreak of bubonic plague[9].

Remember the caterpillars in a cocoon of familiar thinking? Nice cocoon, eh?

Finally, what happens if you actually do end up with rheumatic fever? The only current data we have are from less developed countries where rheumatic fever is still a problem. About 80% of all of these cases occur in children ages 6-15, and the mortality rate is low: between 2-5%. But although it's far from a certain death, between 30-50% of those with rheumatic fever do end up with heart damage (carditis), making prevention a very good idea. Interestingly, once you have rheumatic fever, antibiotic therapy will not prevent heart damage but will only help eradicate the bacteria. It's important to note that eradicating the bacteria is still recommended to prevent further strep infections. None of the other symptoms like rashes, arthritis, etc. from rheumatic fever cause lasting damage.

So let's summarize. A sore throat leads to rheumatic fever only if the sore throat is due to a bacteria in the group A streptococcal family, *and* the person with this strep throat also develops antibodies that cross-react with other proteins in the body, because of their unique genetics. Even then, rheumatic fever is still a very rare event.

Ready to push the envelope and go around the next bend in the river? What if you have a really solid immune system because you sleep well, you eat right, you exercise and when you're at risk of getting sick, you supplement with immune boosters? Since your own immune system is the primary key in fighting off harmful bacteria, doesn't it make sense that having a great immune system could entirely protect you against the strep bacteria? Just chew on that idea for a little bit and if it rattles your cage, take a moment to breathe. This idea may seem shocking if you've been told for your whole life that the only way to be safe from disease is with antibiotics and that there's nothing you can do if you are a victim to other people's sicknesses. Resistance is futile, right? Truly, antibiotics are a fantastic advance and can be really helpful. But they aren't helpful in all situations. In some instances they are overkill or don't work as expected and they always carry side effects. Beyond occasional stomach pain, diarrhea, or nausea, antibiotics wipe out the friendly flora in your gut that is the backbone of your immune system. It's like shooting a cannon ball through your front door to frighten away an intruder. Sure, you might get rid of the intruder, but now you have no front door. I mean, look at the collateral damage!

Finally, please understand that I am certainly not advocating against medical treatment for strep throat. Rather, I want to showcase how our worldviews and beliefs guide our behavior and lead us to faulty conclusions. Magic Bullet thinking would have you believe there is only one option for treatment and one cause for disease when in reality there are multiple treatments and multiple causes.

One last example to showcase Magic Bullet thinking: I heard a news story on NPR about the urge to "find a cure" for Alzheimer's disease by the year 2025. The story talked about funding, of course, and the huge effort being put into research. Not one *second* of the story (at least that I heard) was devoted to the things that we already know have a tremendous preventative impact on Alzheimer's disease: eating right, exercise and learning new things. Instead, we keep looking for yet another Magic Bullet, the one cure that fixes Alzheimer's no matter how many supersized burgers and fries we are downing.

A More Realistic Alternative to Magic Bullets

The approach in *The Fix* is not about Magic Bullets. There's no one magic supplement, pharmaceutical medication, herbal tea or other treatment that will make all your problems go away.

Instead, reality is about multiple streams of interacting cause and effect. Like I said in the introduction, you can't just start taking holy basil for your Type II Diabetes without making any other changes and expect a full recovery. It's not because holy basil is no good; it's because your lifestyle flows like the Mississippi River, and one little addition or subtraction isn't nearly enough to change the course of that river. On the other hand, if you are tackling the big stuff in your health by eating right, sleeping right and exercising, the addition of a particular supplement or treatment may have a much more palpable effect. If you are already affecting the course of your river in a huge way with the right food, sleep and exercise, then your body is better able to benefit from a judicious application of other helps.

Let me illustrate further with a car analogy:

The Mustang Analogy

You have this 2002 Mustang in the garage and even though it's a great car, it just won't run. You take it to your trusted mechanic and he reads the engine code on his computer that says you need a new oxygen sensor. So you replace the oxygen sensor, but the car still doesn't work. Back to the mechanic. This time he says it needs new spark plugs. So you get new spark plugs... and the car still doesn't run. (Sound familiar, anyone?) You take it back to the mechanic. Again. Third time's the charm, right? Now he says it's a vacuum leak. So you get that fixed. And still the car won't work.

At this point you're thinking you need a new mechanic! All those wasted dollars replacing parts that weren't even the actual problem!

So next you take your car to a new guy, a high-tech mechanic that your friend recommended to you. This guy listens to what you've been through and says that you have a dirty mass airflow sensor. He fixes that. Now the car runs like it should.[f]

The issue here is not that the first mechanic was wrong and the second mechanic found the actual problem. In reality, all of those issues were real, valid problems. The parts that were fixed prior to the mass airflow sensor all needed to be fixed. Just fixing the mass airflow sensor alone would not have done the trick. But with Magic Bullet thinking, we tend to look for

---

[f]Thanks to my brother, John, for help with this analogy.

one problem and one solution. The fact is, we have multiple problems and multiple solutions and we need to incorporate all those solutions in order to "run right."

Similarly, it doesn't make a lot of sense to go searching from specialist to specialist for the one answer that will finally do the trick. It's probable that there are multiple things that are wrong and you will need more than one solution.

This is the alternative to Magic Bullet thinking: looking at multiple causes and multiple solutions. If it helps, try viewing this alternative as *systems thinking* rather than the linear thinking of Magic Bullet.

Systems thinking looks at the whole picture and sees how little things in one area influence little things in another area, and how these further set off other little things that in turn create a breeding ground for current problems. Systems are complex and contain multiple paths, multiple directions and multiple outcomes. Often fixing one or two things won't be enough for real change. But this doesn't mean that those one or two things don't need to be fixed. Rather, it just means that you need to do more, try more, and fix more instead of giving in or giving up.

You can't just start drinking spinach every morning without changing your 1200 calorie lunchtime habits. Spinach will help you, sure, but it won't overcome a supersized cheeseburger, fries and a large chocolate shake.

Systems thinking assumes that the system seeks *homeostasis*, or in other words, balance. Similarly, a holistic view of health assumes that the body naturally works toward wellness. The body's responses to problems are seen as a path toward healing. For example, fever is the body's response to illness and it raises body temperature high enough to kill pathogens.

Stuck in Magic Bullet Thinking

We know that there are behaviors we can do to raise or lower our risk for various illnesses, but our society remains stuck in Magic Bullet thinking. Our system of getting scientifically based treatments is stuck in Magic Bullet thinking as well. For example, instead of understanding how vitamin D might make our whole system work better, we run a randomized controlled trial looking at vitamin D versus a placebo and its effect on some disease.[g] If Vitamin D isn't shown to improve that particular disease it's concluded that we are wasting our time when we take that supplement. In fact, the situation just might be just like the spark plugs on that Mustang. Perhaps there are other things needed to resolve the disease *along with* sufficient vitamin D. There are effective ways to study this, but when scientists are stuck in Magic Bullet thinking, they are very unlikely to realize they haven't included all the important variables in their experiment.

---

[g] Just before publishing this book, I saw an example of this exact scenario, published in the Lancet (11 October 2013). The discussion centered on how Vitamin D doesn't help bone density and therefore may be a waste of time. Perfect real-life example of what I'm talking about!

Symptom-Focused Thinking

Even worse, instead of solving the underlying problem, much of our medical thinking focuses on resolving symptoms. By relieving symptoms we somehow believe we have gotten rid of the problem.

Perhaps one of the most egregious examples of the symptom focused approach is cholesterol lowering medications. The purpose of these medications is to reduce heart disease, the foundational idea being that high cholesterol leads to heart disease. However, data show fairly clearly that high cholesterol is not the primary cause of heart disease, but instead a symptom. So lowering cholesterol may not be the answer. Rather, we should seek to understand why cholesterol is unnaturally high. Treating the symptom in this case does not treat the cause, and if you treat the symptom with statin drugs, you are signing up for a whole lot of dangerous side effects in addition to not treating the cause!

You may have heard some time ago that eating fat is bad and raises your cholesterol. Then perhaps you heard that the link between dietary fat and heart disease is pretty weak. Your best friend tells you eggs are bad for you and the next day your aunt shares an article saying eggs are healthy. But your doctor still urges you to eat a low-fat diet. Magic Bullet thinking just leaves you confused with all this information and you start to wonder whom to trust. You get cynical and you just want to throw up your hands and give up. Nobody knows what will help, so you might as well enjoy yourself and chomp down that cheeseburger, right?

Holistic thinking puts all of this into a larger context. That larger context can help you make more sense of what you read and hear about many health issues. Let's look more closely at the fat vs. heart disease problem, and examine how context can change what we see.

A recent meta-analysis (a sophisticated way of pooling study results) looked at studies examining saturated fat and heart disease, and found that increased intake of saturated fat was not related to increased risk of cardiovascular disease.[10] But wait, this doesn't mean go break out the butter and have a party! Let's zoom out a little more and find a bigger picture.

Studies that look at fat intake in the standard American diet may suffer from what statisticians call a *restriction of range* problem. This is to say, there is not enough of a difference in fat intake among the population to explain our significant differences in heart disease. A "low-fat" diet in America is far different from a "low-fat" diet in China. Rather than saying fat intake doesn't matter because there are no visible differences in people's health whether they are consuming a 29% fat diet (the percentage of fat in the average American low fat diet) or a 37% fat diet (the percentage of fat in the average American diet), let's zoom out a bit more and think about how the American diet compares to the average diet in China.

A high-fat diet in China contains less fat than the American low-fat diet. The percentage of fat in the average high-fat Chinese diet is just 24% fat. The Chinese low fat diet is only 6% fat. In this example you see that all Americans eat a relatively high-fat diet. So it makes more sense that it's hard to see a difference in heart disease outcomes between two groups that are more similar to each other than they are different. The point here is not about fat percentages, but about seeing the facts from a different vantage point. Context is crucial.

A Cascade of Causation

When we talk about the connection between physical and emotional health, we often get stuck looking at symptoms rather than at the big picture. For instance, we look at how certain physical diseases affect our emotional health. As one example, people with multiple sclerosis often experience depression and not just the "I hate this disease and it's depressing" kind of depression. Emotionally healthy people with MS experience depression more frequently than people without MS. In fact, some neurologists routinely prescribe an antidepressant at the same time they make the initial diagnosis. This approach, looking at how various physical illnesses affect emotional health does have a good deal of merit, and we certainly need to know what substances affect what condition. But it's more complicated than that.

Let's think about Maxine again. A low thyroid and Lyme disease are both associated with depression. They are connected. But the connection is more than just one thing causing another. It's not a game of low thyroid + Lyme = depression, so fix the thyroid and Lyme and the depression will go away. There's a reason that Maxine has Lyme disease and it's not just because she might have been bitten by a tick. It also has to do with her immune system, which has to do with her sleeping, eating and exercise habits which are influenced by how she feels. And those sleeping, eating and exercise habits also exert influence back the other way, resulting in how she feels. Add her history of ear infections (and subsequent antibiotic treatment), long-term gastrointestinal problems, irregular menses, and you start to approach a complicated reality. This reality is similar to the problems many of us face. These challenges are complicated, multi-directional and have more than one cause and more than one outcome. So while medical science may focus on specific conditions, you need to understand that this narrow focus is in many ways artificial. It is done out of convenience. Real people in real situations are far more complex, and we need to understand and remember that one thing leads to another.

It's time to shell out for the whole package: sparkplugs to mass airflow sensor.

You can't expect to fix your cold virus and the fact that you are getting a cold four or five times a year, yet still eat sugary cereal for breakfast, burgers and fries for lunch, and stay up late every weekend. Listen to your body and listen well. It will tell you what you need to notice and do.

The Whole Is Greater

Your body is a whole, and the parts are not ignorant of each other. Stress affects your blood sugar as does lack of exercise. Lack of exercise affects your stress. All of these create inflammation which might lead to irritable bowel symptoms or perhaps heart disease. The donuts and burgers will help that along nicely! One thing leads to another, multiple things lead to multiple outcomes, and you find yourself in a spiral that feels out of control.

One thing leads to another in terms of fixing problems too. Improving one area of your health can help you become more resistant to stress of all kinds. For example, if you correct your blood sugar issue, life looks better. If you can get a reduction in stress hormones, you'll feel better still. If you have decent nutrition, you feel even better. Life seems more manageable after a good night's sleep. Maybe teenage daughters are challenge for anyone, but you can manage them a whole lot better if you're physically intact. You *can* get out of the death spiral. Just stay with me and I'll help you make the changes you need in order to stop spinning.

Life — the whole complex package — is a challenge. To live the challenge of life while physically "down" is like hiking Mount Everest with a brick in your pack. It's hard enough without the brick[h]. Let's *Fix* that!

---

[h] Another great line from Dr. Stephenson!

Chapter Four

Empiricism is for Open Minds

E mpiricism is for folks with open minds. You'll see what I mean.

First, data are just data. In other words, numbers or information don't have their own meaning, rather, they have the meaning we assign them. They are only meaningful in context, and context is what *we* bring. We assign data a meaning based on what else we know, what else is going on, and what we think. Consider the example of the "low-fat" diet we just talked about. It's all about context. Data are interpreted as part of a previously arranged context that grows from who we are, what we believe, and what we are predicting.

Empiricism is a method of getting knowledge. Basically when you ask "How do you know that?" a person who uses the empirical method will tell you "I know because I watched it happen," or "I took a picture and here it is," or "Here are fifty people who saw it happen." You can contrast this method with *authoritarianism* which uses an authority to tell you what knowledge is ("I know because Dr. Authority said so."), or *pragmatism* ("It's practical so it's right."), or *rationalism* ("I know it's true because it is a result of logic."). These four particular ways of knowing are some of the favorites in our society, but at this point in time we especially love empiricism. Scientists rely on empiricism as their primary method for gaining knowledge or identifying truths. Research methodology (how people set up a research study) uses the empirical method to find out what *is*. At least that's the underlying intent of empirical research.

> *Our biases compromise our ability to interpret data....it's awfully hard to have a truly open mind because we grow up steeped in what we think we know about the world.*

In the current health care climate we are seeing a real struggle between two factions: the natural health care advocates and conventional medicine. Sometimes the struggle gets so polarized it feels like a war. This is most unfortunate because both "sides" have a lot to contribute and could learn from one another. Each side has its thoughtful supporters and its rabid rabble rousers, its true believers and dispassionate hopefuls. Each side looks down at the other side across a field littered with suffering human bodies. Although there are some health professionals who attempt to sit in the middle, most of these operate more out of a desire for eclectic efficiency rather than from an underlying, comprehensive model of understanding. That is to say, there are any number of clinicians who call themselves integrative but who use a cafeteria approach as a means of treating their patients. What makes them integrative in their own minds is merely that their "treatment cafeteria" serves both allopathic and alternative medicines. Integrative care in this sense is simply picking and choosing from an à la carte menu.

Thinking about it, you may realize that this attempt at an integrative approach is still served up Magic Bullet style, whether or not the bullet looks like a herb or was made by a pharmaceutical company. Illness, diagnosis, cure, all better. It's pretty fortunate for most people that this simple approach can still, at times, work pretty well in the short-term.

Nobody Is Winning

I want to make it extremely clear that not only are there *not* merely two sides on the current health scene, but that neither of these apparent sides have all the truth. Both have their share of dedicated, thoughtful doctors, both have their share of charlatans and abusers of power and both sides have their share of incompetent clinicians whose thinking may not be lucid or accurate, and who seek safety in sticking to the party line. When we get fooled into swallowing an either/or style of thinking, we compromise our ability to think clearly about facts. We feel pressured to hold to a party line; the result is that our biases compromise our ability to interpret data.

We See Through a Dark Glass (Bias)

Empiricism is simply a way of knowing things either by looking at facts, or by doing experiments or both. Empiricism works best when what we believe does not influence the experiments or the results; that way the facts can be interpreted on their own merits. Thus, empiricism is for folks with open minds. The inherent weakness in the empirical approach is this: It's awfully, awfully hard to have a truly open mind! We grow up steeped in what we think we know about the world.

Interestingly, some recent evidence points to the fascinating ability we humans have to literally change our minds (as in our *brains!*) in response to social pressure. A recent article in *Science* examined the memories of people who were pressured by others to believe something that was inaccurate. Turns out that people responded to this pressure by agreeing to the "party line." But here's where it gets interesting: Once the study members caved into believing something that wasn't true, the researchers found through brain scans that physical traces of participants' memories of the true facts were actually changed, even when the initial memory had been strong and accurate![11] Studies like this highlight how the interaction between bias and interpretation of data in the search for scientific truth is fraught with complications.

One of the casualties of the war between natural health care and conventional medicine is knowledge. Rather than understanding what we see, differing sides are grabbing hold of data and forcing the data to mean what they want. They are narrowing the context used to interpret the data, whether consciously or unconsciously. But data don't take sides. They are just the data. It is people who are responsible for the interpretations made based on beliefs and experiences. We bring the context.

Most people believe in what they call "medical science." But by this, they generally mean what they read in magazines or newspapers that's written by experts, what they see on television or the internet, or what their friends or doctors tell them as fact. So when they say that they know something, what they are usually saying is that they heard it from someone they consider to be a good authority.

So where does the authority get his or her information? Certainly that authority's accumulated professional education can provide some good answers. When physicians have questions that go beyond their medical training, studies show that most of them consult a combination of online resources based on scientific articles (for example, the online site UpToDate), medical textbooks or their colleagues[12,13]. Services that offer seminars or other kinds of continuing education are additional sources of knowledge; these sources also draw from studies published in medical journals.

What most of us in the general public believe is that medical practitioners, researchers, medical reporters, etc. are all relying on scientific data. Certainly that is what medical professionals are looking for when they read publications in medical journals. This is called empirical data, and most of us believe that medical journals report actual empirical data. But generally medical journals report the results of medical studies already interpreted for their readers in a ready-made context. Scientists have shaped a story out of their data long before it's published, and this story depends on what they believe about how the world works.

How can there not be polarization between those (generally academics) who seem to worship exclusively at the "altar" of the scientific method and those who, disgusted with the current state of science, have thrown out the entire method and claim to "not believe in science." (Unfortunately, the natural health world has a lot of these kinds of practitioners.)

The scientific method is not to blame. The method works if you follow it. It's just that the method is often not followed very well.

Ways of Knowing

To further illustrate how we think we "know" things, let's examine the Mediterranean diet (a way of eating that includes lots of fruits, vegetables, nuts, whole grains, fish, and olives or olive oil) and some of the different ways we might know whether this diet is good for you...

...says Dr. Oz (this is authoritarianism).

...because we know the components are good for us, so overall it makes sense (this is rationalism).

...because we've experienced that it helps people get healthier (this is pragmatism).

...because a study conducted in 2009[14] showed that people who adhered to this diet were up to 30% less likely to develop depression, had a lower risk for stroke and were less likely to develop Alzheimer's disease (this is empiricism).

Let's look at another example: how we think we know whether dietary fat is good for us.

We all "know" fat is bad for us. We should all eat a low-fat diet. We've known this for decades, right? I remember the pride I felt in the late 1980's as I cooked super low-fat food for my family. But wait, what was this "knowledge" based on? Supermarket magazines? Things your Home Economics teacher told you? Dare I say it – things your *doctor* told you?

Cooking low fat food merely because that's all you have available is an example of pragmatism. In this case you're being practical and using what's on hand.

If, however, the reason you have no fat available to cook with is because you have logically concluded that when you eat fat, you get fat, you are using rationalism as your way of knowing the truth. Here, for purposes of illustrating rationalism, we're ignoring the fact that your conclusions are wrong! Thinking rationally doesn't mean that your assumptions are correct, it just requires that you logically derive your reasons.

But most likely, you eat low fat because you believe experts have told you that you should. This is authoritarianism.

Do you know what empirical data show about dietary fats?

There are good and bad fats. Eating good fats (these include nuts, seeds, fish, olive oil, avocados and even leafy green vegetables – what!? yes, leafy greens have fat in them!) lowers your risk of depression[15] and eating bad fats (trans fats) raises your depression risk... and your stroke risk... and your cancer risk. What the empirical data support is not eating low fat, but rather eliminating the *trans fats* you'd find in many donuts, burgers, fried foods (yes, essentially all your pleasurable sources of fat. Sorry.) These data have been around for years, but many still believe they are virtuous when they eat fat-free. Incidentally, coconut oil is a great example of a healthy fat that has been vilified for decades. The empirical evidence is that coconut oil (2 tablespoons per day) not only helps men and women lose inches on their waists, but it also boosts HDL cholesterol (the "good" kind of cholesterol).[16]

So eating fat can be good for you, if you eat the right kinds of fats. In fact, you need to eat fats in order to achieve optimum health! Fats are crucial to your cell functioning, your brain functioning, and your body's ability to send nutrients from one area to another. Distinguishing between good and bad fats is a significantly different approach than simply eliminating all sources of fat.

What we're talking about here is empiricism. Empirical knowledge is simply knowledge that is obtained through observation and study: "I see it therefore I know it."

But seeing involves interpreting, and, as we have been illustrating, therein lies the problem.

Conventional medicine versus alternative medicine has become a confusing and ineffective battle of opposing lines. Loyalty to the party has outstripped folks' ability to interpret the data objectively.

Manipulation: Shameless and Subtle

Here's one extreme example of how one side of this debate can shamelessly manipulate an audience. A fairly recent internet article about eradicating feral pigs in Michigan reads "mass murder spree of pigs of the wrong color" and "racial profiling for animal murder," and includes the subheading "Got the wrong hair color? The state of Michigan will kill you." Although the website writers changed some of their particularly offensive language soon after publication, the original article included the phrase "Michigan to kill all blacks" as a heading (shown in this website, copied from the original website the day the article was released.[i] The article on the original website was quickly toned down to remove this language). This kind of biased thinking and writing is typical of extremists, and unfortunately what happens is that many people react by disbelieving everything such sources have ever said or written rather than rejecting

[i] Accessed March 30, 2012.
  http://www.ar15.com/forums/t_1_5/1304957_.html
The modified article can be found at
  http://www.naturalnews.com/035372_Michigan_pigs_farm_freedom.html, accessed March 30, 2012.

merely that one questionable article. Here's one reason why this tends to happen: When we feel disgust or other strong emotions, our brain tends to make us think more categorically, or in "all or nothing" terms. Our extreme reactions lead us to "throw out the baby with the bathwater." Sometimes our emotional reactions yield good results, but thinking emotionally instead of rationally can be dangerous.

Similarly, less blatant proponents of one camp or the other can push us more subtly (and therefore more insidiously). A headline in the LA Times[j] reads "Dietary supplements risky for older women, study finds" and the article's first line tells us that "An increased risk of death is seen in those who took multivitamins, folic acid, iron and others." Right away you're thinking about stopping any of those multivitamins or other supplements you might be taking. However, a look at the original scientific publication[17] that this article is based on reveals the bias. Data from the actual publication just doesn't support these pithy headline interpretations, and one is left wondering who wants women to stop taking vitamins.

Not only did this newspaper article sensationalize the original study's findings, but a closer look at the scientific publication itself[18] revealed damaging weaknesses in the methodology and design of the study itself. Two fairly large problems loomed. The first was that the study assumed all supplements are of equal

[j]http://articles.latimes.com/2011/oct/10/health/la-he-vitamins, accessed March 30, 2012

quality. The quality of a supplement can transform how the body reacts to it. The second problem was that it looks possible that women who were included in the initial data collection as non-supplement users could have then started taking supplements in the final year of the study (18 years later) and then have been classified as supplement users in the final analysis. In other words, a woman could have taken no supplements for 17 years of the study, then started taking supplements in that last year (perhaps because she discovered a serious problem?) yet still be counted as part of the supplement-taking group. I think it's an irresponsible leap to distort the findings of this study into a frightening headline declaring that supplements might cause death in older women.

We Are Cocooned in Bias

Hopefully, the foregoing examples have highlighted for you the greatest challenge to relying on empirical data: interpretation of that data. We can only look at the data from where we sit, and we all sit inside a pervasive world of bias. Most people interpret data according to whether or not it supports their points of view (confirmatory bias) rather than on the merits alone of the data, and what these data might mean outside of their preconceived notions of the world.

You are now probably wondering how it's ever possible to figure out what is true and real given these inherent problems in the empirical method, not to mention the additional challenges of ferreting out what's true and real in the atmosphere of bickering between adherents of

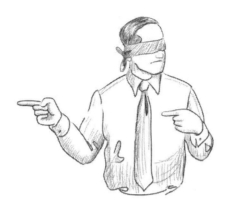

either allopathic or alternative medicine. Since both sides contain vocal groups who are passionate and well-meaning about their beliefs, it's unsettling to recognize that some ideas you may have considered to be "medical science" may not be entirely accurate.

This book can't offer you any magic reveals or guaranteed roads to Real Factual Knowledge. All I can do is try to shed some light on the problem and advise that you become your own empiricist. Try things out for yourself. Use your knowledge and mind as best as you can to gather all the information you can find. Make the best decisions possible based on what you know. Ask experts, but be aware of bias. Put a solution into play and then gather your own data. Evaluate your results. Refine your solution and repeat as necessary. This is the second Big Idea in this book:

> ## *Big Idea#2*
> *Empiricism is not only for folks with open minds, but also for folks with courage. Have the courage to find out, experiment with what works for you, and take charge of your own health.*

Not long ago, I was listening to a podcast about the perils of pop psychology and how people would use what they thought of as psychologically sound common sense to solve their problems, only to find out that such "pop psychology" principles were totally unsupported by the data. One example given – and this example has been one of my favorites to debunk in therapy for over a decade – is the idea that we think it is healthy for us to act angry when we feel angry. That is to say, we believe that "getting it out" is necessary and makes sense. I've seen this idea supported in all kinds of treatment facilities from encouraging inmates to "get out" their aggression through exercising all the way to telling children that they should pound pillows when they are frustrated.[k]

Most people think that this is a psychologically helpful idea and that getting anger "out" will make them more emotionally sound. But it actually backfires because what you are doing when you try to "get out" your

---

[k] Here's a really great article discussing this myth and its history. http://www.psychologicalscience.org/media/myths/myth_30.cfm

anger is merely practicing being angry. Guess what happens next time you're angry? You're better at acting angry![19] You've achieved a new norm. This is a great example of how one pop psychology myth proves really unhelpful. It's also an example of how we think we know truth, when what we know is actually myth.

But here's the thing: being skeptical is not necessarily the same thing as being open-minded to what the data actually say. Many skeptics pride themselves on their supposed empiricism, but in the earlier mentioned radio show I also heard skeptics bashing acupuncture and touch therapy as being absolutely ridiculous. It was strongly implied that these were two treatments entirely unsupported by any scientific data, and that only a crackpot would engage in such treatments. No actual data about these treatments was discussed. Here is skepticism, yes, but had it been supported with any empirical data? The truth is that the body of acupuncture knowledge has quite a bit of empirical support[1]. Touch therapy finds fairly limited support, but there are some data that indicate touch therapy might be helpful. This example shows how the problem of bias includes gleeful skeptics who in their rush to be skeptical, fail to be open-minded to data.

I'd like to point out as strongly as I can this truth: Data don't take sides.

Empirical science is an equal opportunity employer. If you create a solid and unbiased

---

[1] Of course it has had thousands of years of observational support in China!

research design, the data will represent what happens. Data won't care if you are Republican or Democrat, purple or blue, male or mushroom. Data don't take sides.

The problem is that unbiased research designs simply don't exist. Since our understanding of the world is a work in progress, we will always be limited. We can only become more aware of our own biases and how they create the glasses we use to view the world.

My goal in writing this book is not to help natural medicine or allopathic medicine to "win." My goal is simply to help people feel better, act better and live better.

Chapter Five

Three-Legged Stool

One of the few bridges we have between the two worlds of conventional medicine and alternative medicine is the growing and undeniable reality of the mind body connection.

To a certain extent we all know that the way we think affects how we feel, both physically and mentally. Emotions play a part in what we think about, emotions play a part in our health, and our thoughts affect our emotions.

One of the purposes of this book is to emphasize that these connections are more profound than most of us realize, and that they affect us on a deeper and more day-to-day and moment-to-moment manner than perhaps we yet understand.

The mind-body connection is far more pervasive than we traditionally think. Take a look at the graphically illustrated traditional understanding (the top half of the diagram).

We are comfortable acknowledging that our minds can affect our bodies, and vice versa. However most of us don't fathom how deeply these connections go. Mind and body are so merged that their separation at all is mostly a convenience for our thinking. (Note how the words mind and body are merged in the lower circle.)

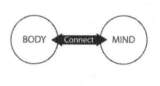

Even very casual glances at the current medical literature show that most scientists consider it pretty obvious that our thoughts and emotions profoundly affect our bodies (and our health) and that the functioning of our bodies profoundly affects our thoughts and emotions. As a quick illustration, did you know that a study found that people become more impatient when they see fast-food logos, even when they see them unconsciously? Not only does impatience increase, but people start showing a preference for anything that saves time (like combined shampoo and conditioner) and they want immediate rewards![20]

What I'm saying to you, practically speaking, is that all that discouragement and all those donuts are far more linked than you may think! And, I can help you with BOTH.

Myths, Skeptics and Ignorance

I was listening to a medical radio show in which the host was discussing gastrointestinal disorders. A caller asked about swallowing petroleum jelly to help with ulcerative colitis. Alarmed (and frankly, disgusted) I turned up the volume, to better hear the gastroenterologist's reply. He soundly rejected the petroleum jelly solution (thank goodness! I mean, America runs on petroleum products, but really?). He then lumped all non-pharmaceutical solutions together in one fell swoop, saying that there were no home remedies or homeopathic solutions that would be able to help with ulcerative colitis, except, maybe (and he said this snidely as if it were an outlandish and extremist notion) healthy eating, and he went on to discuss the current conventional medical approach to this problem. I sat there, my mouth open in amazement as I heard this expert openly admit that healthy eating would resolve a problem that creates untold misery for close to a million Americans, and then proceed to sweep that cost-effective, realistic and beneficial solution under the rug in favor of more complicated, more expensive and less effective solutions.

Not only that, this was a great example of how so many people equate all forms of complementary and alternative medicine (CAM) as essentially the same kind of "thing." You know, the "thing" where homeopathic medicine means anything from chiropractic help for your back, to mindfulness practice for depression, to, well, petroleum jelly for ulcerative colitis.

So perhaps before we go on, we should do a

quick fix in this area. Here are a few definitions to help you understand some terms from the world of holistic health:

CAM refers to ***Complementary and Alternative medicine***. This is essentially any form of medicine that is not Western or conventional/allopathic medicine and includes everything from therapeutic pets to reiki to chiropractic to homeopathy to herbal medicine. It's a huge category. Using this term is like dividing the world's music resources into classical music (conventional medicine) and everything else (CAM).

Herbal and homeopathic medicines are two branches of alternative medicine that seem to be most often confused. Herbal medicine and homeopathic medicine are not the same thing. ***Herbal medicine*** is the use of plants to help heal the body or promote well-being in the body. ***Homeopathic medicine*** is directed to helping the body feel better but doesn't use whole herbs in the same manner as does herbal medicine. Homeopathic remedies are made by systematically diluting substances and then applying those diluted substances based on the theory of opposites[m].

Acupuncture, massage therapy, chiropractic practice, meditation, energy therapy, Ayurvedic medicine and Traditional Chinese Medicine (TCM) are likely the most popular forms of CAM in addition to herbal medicine and homeopathic medicine. Each of these forms of healing must be understood on its own within the

---

[m]A complete discussion is beyond the scope of this book.

context of how that system views illness, or "disease" and how it proposes to bring the body back to health. Likewise, and this is very important, research that examines these methods must be conducted by investigators who understand how their methods must operate within each specific healing system in order to attain valid results. For example, giving fifteen minute massages right before chemotherapy and then measuring whether or not a group with massages did better than a group without massages is not a good measure of the efficacy of massage therapy as a whole. It is only a test of how well a 15 minute massage right before chemotherapy acts. (In my opinion, this example resembles doing a study on whether or not a kiss on the cheek before being punched in the face makes you feel better about being punched). Similarly, taking the local drugstore chain's version of a multivitamin and probiotic combination is not likely to tell you much about how useful vitamins or probiotics in general might be. Rather, it will just tell you how useful that drugstore chain's pill is likely to be.

Home remedies don't really fit into any one of these categories, as they are usually remedies based on folk wisdom, relying on items most people have around the house. Some may have their roots in one or more of the above CAM or conventional treatments. For example, using powdered alum to treat a canker sore or using baking soda to settle an upset stomach are both effective home remedies that are understandable given the underlying chemistry involved.

It's important to not confuse these varying systems of healing and make the mistake of either assuming that success in one equals legitimacy for all, or vice versa. When CAM is viewed (as is often the case in current American medical culture) as *any* alternative to conventional medicine, and then treated as if any one form is just as good (or nutty) as another as it was in the radio show above (remember – "home remedies or any other kind of homeopathic treatment") you and a host of others are losing a whole lot of information and a great deal of potential help.

Here's another way of illustrating my point that it's unwise to lump all modalities of alternative healing together as equally effective or ineffective: It's as if I thought of carbohydrates as any food other than fat or animal products (meat, eggs, dairy). In this kind of thinking, a serving of broccoli would be carbs, a serving of donuts could be carbs, and a serving of potatoes likewise would be considered as carbs.

Oh, wait. We do think that way in America.

Three-legged Stool: A Foundation for Whole Health

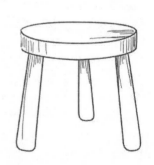

There are three things I ask all my patients to do – three things that are a foundation for whole health. Just like a three-legged stool, these three things provide a solid foundation that is hard to tip over.

When my patients fix these three things, a remarkable thing happens: at least some and sometimes all or nearly all of their psychological problems disappear.

These three things aren't special, novel or shocking in any way. You already know what they are: eating, sleeping and exercise. You probably got sick to death of your mother telling you to do these three things. But perhaps you don't quite appreciate just how important they are, or the extent of their far reaching effects.

I don't think it's a coincidence that most of America suffers from enormous sleep debt, horrifying eating practices and a stunning lack of exercise, while at the same time Americans are experiencing ever-increasing levels of illness, including psychiatric illnesses. I'm a little dumbfounded when people seem mystified by the increase in health problems like heart disease, diabetes and depression. These problems are connected to our foundational health through our eating, sleeping and exercise habits. It's Big Idea Number Three.

> *Big Idea #3:*
> *Eating, sleeping and exercise habits*
> *are the three-legged stool*
> *your overall health rests on.*

Chapter Six

Making Food Your Medicine

The average person in America eats 2700 calories per day, far more than is needed for an average person. The physical and psychological cost of not only overeating but of *what* we are eating is staggering. The current food pyramid indicates that a person who eats 2000 calories per day should include 9 servings of fruits and vegetables (that's 4 and 1/2 cups — and lettuce and other leafy greens are measured such that you need to eat 2 cups of lettuce in order for it to count as a 1 cup serving of vegetables). Some Americans eat only corn or potatoes (or ketchup) as vegetables, usually in the form of chips or fries.

The diet I advocate for, as better for your whole heath, is one that is rich in plants and sparing in animal products. If you can obtain about half your total calories from vegetables, no more than 10% from animal products or sweets, and the rest from fruits, nuts, seeds and grains, I think you'll enjoy significantly improved overall health. This chapter focuses on why I think a plant-based diet makes sense.

Diet and Emotions:
A Vegetarian Diet Might Improve your Mood

I have been interested in the impact of food on mood for over twenty years. Here's a recent study that I think is pretty interesting.

Researchers compared people who were relatively healthy eaters and who stuck to either a vegetarian diet or to an omnivore diet. They found that vegetarians reported fewer negative emotions than omnivores[21]. Furthermore, the vegetarian eaters had significantly lower levels of EPA and DHA (essential fatty acids) as compared to the omnivores. This was interesting because the scientific literature has found that on average, people with higher levels of EPA and DHA enjoy a happier mood. But in this study, vegetarians had fewer negative emotions despite their lower levels of these essential fatty acids.

So the researchers did a follow-up study – a randomized controlled trial this time. They asked people who were all omnivores and who ate meat at least once per day to participate. The individuals were divided into three groups. For two weeks one group ate the omnivore diet (meat at least once each day), one group ate a fish based diet (fish three or four times per week, no meat or poultry but eggs and dairy were fine), and the third group ate a vegetarian diet that included dairy products. Essential fatty acid levels of the participants were measured before and after the study. Even though the group that ate a vegetarian diet showed decreased EPA and DHA levels after the two week period, this group showed an *improvement* in mood. And although the people in the fish eating group showed an increase of 100% in their levels of EPA and DHA, they did not experience improvement in mood. So although these particular volunteers had not been leading a vegetarian lifestyle, nor did they particularly believe in vegetarian philosophies, they still enjoyed a decline in general anxiety and psychological distress after just two weeks of a lacto-vegetarian diet. The study concluded that vegetarians "may cope better with mental stress than omnivores"[22].

> *Just a side note here -- In the Old Testament, the God Jehovah commanded the children of Israel to eat bitter herbs right after spending some time contemplating the pain of their Egyptian captivity. This was part of the Passover ritual. Modern-day Jews who observe Passover still continue this ritual. We also know that bitter herbs serve to help the liver function better. I don't think this is a coincidence. Pass the parsley.*

More Nutrients

A primarily vegetarian diet includes far more nutrition than a primarily meat-based diet. Also, we know that animal products increase inflammation (in part because they raise levels of arachidonic acid) and we know that inflammation is associated with negative mood states. Indeed, the researchers in this study brought inflammation up as one explanation for their results.

What I also find interesting here is that studies like these turn the Magic Bullet style of thinking on its head. Achieving better mood is more than merely popping pills, even if they are EPA and DHA pills. There is something bigger and more complex happening when we make the switch to a mostly plant-based diet[n].

Food Is More Than Fuel

Only a few years ago many physicians were convinced that what you ate had almost nothing to do with your health, as long as you consumed sufficient vitamins and minerals. At present, most people now know that eating more vegetables and less processed or fast foods can have a significant impact on your vulnerability to disease.

But why are plant foods good for us?

All plants use the process of photosynthesis to produce three products necessary for their growth and development: carbohydrates, proteins and fats (and their inherent vitamins and minerals). We call these three products the plant's *primary metabolites*. It may surprise you to learn that the romaine

---

[n] A plant based diet is not always the same thing as a vegetarian diet. You can eat a "vegetarian" diet that is based in toaster pastries, peanut butter sandwiches and macaroni and soy cheese. Technically you are vegetarian, but you are eating a pretty unhealthy diet that doesn't include many actual vegetables.

lettuce in your salad has fat in it, or that the potato on your plate is a source of protein, but it's true.

Plants use carbohydrates for structure (cellulose is a carbohydrate) and energy (glucose is a carbohydrate). Humans also use carbohydrates for energy, but we don't use cellulose. We can't even digest it because we lack the enzymes necessary to break it down. The cellulose we eat is what we call fiber, and despite the fact we can't digest it, it's necessary for a properly functioning intestinal tract. What we actually digest from plants are simple and complex sugars like glucose and starch. We use these carbohydrates as primary energy sources in order to protect our body's store of protein.

Plants use fats (also called lipids) to create their cell membranes, to store energy, and to transmit information between cells. We humans use fats in the same way. We don't usually think of plants as having fats, but plants, in fact, produce "the majority of the world's lipids and most animals, including humans, depend on these lipids as a major source of calories and essential fatty acids."[23]

Wait a moment! What are essential fatty acids?

Essential fatty acids are fats that our bodies can't produce on our own. Our bodies can modify some of the fats we eat and use them to create other fats that we need, but only to a certain extent. There are some fats we cannot make that are crucial to our survival. These fats are therefore called *essential* because we can't make them from other raw materials. We have to ingest them.

Essential fatty acids ultimately come from plants. Even if we eat animal flesh that contains these fats, the fats originally came from plants.

Plants also need proteins just like all living things. Proteins are critical to the structure, function and regulation of cells in plants as well as in humans. The building blocks for protein are amino acids. Think of proteins as chains of amino acids. Of the many amino acids discovered, there are 22 amino acids that are critical to human health. Of these 22, our body can manufacture 13. This leaves 9 that we can't manufacture on our own. We name these nine "essential amino acids" just like we have named the fats we can't manufacture in the body "essential fatty acids."

Plants are the ultimate, original source of protein. Animals eat plants and concentrate that plant protein in their body tissues, but the protein itself comes originally from plants. Not all plants contain all of the amino acids, and many plants don't contain all of the nine essential

Secondary metabolites

vary, depending on the plant and region in question. Each plant type has a unique mixture of many of these secondary metabolites.

Secondary metabolites perform a variety of functions, including acting to help defend the plant from destruction or helping attract pollinators (smell, color and pattern, flavor, etc.). There are thousands of new secondary metabolites discovered each year. We know of over 100,000 secondary metabolites. Secondary metabolites are the sources of a plant's medicinal qualities or other unique effects. Caffeine and morphine are two examples.

amino acids. But ingesting food from a variety of plant sources (for example, black beans and corn) will easily provide all nine essential amino acids.

When you think of food as merely fats, proteins and carbohydrates — the primary metabolites — you are missing much of what creates good nutrition. Food that's nourishing for you contains much more than the primary metabolites, even if you ingest your full complement of vitamins and minerals. Plants also produce *secondary metabolites*°, which are biologically active substances that can help us with a host of positive cellular activities in the body. You can think of the action of plant secondary metabolites in your body as comparable to how the same secondary metabolites work in the actual plant. They are not critical for growth, but instead are used to help the plant interact with the world in a way that promotes health — both for the plant and for those of us who eat that plant.

Here's an analogy to help you understand what I'm saying: Having a studio apartment is like having your physical life's basics taken care of. You have a kitchen area, a sleeping area, a bathroom area — just like having your necessary fats, proteins and carbohydrates. Anything extra like a dishwasher or wall hanging is like the plant's secondary metabolites. You can survive on basics, but your quality of life really depends on ingesting more nutrients than just the bare bones — fats, proteins and carbohydrates.

° Secondary metabolites also go by the term phytonutrients.

You may have heard of some of these plant secondary metabolites without realizing what they were. Here are some examples:

Flavonoids are plant pigments, but ingesting flavonoids is not at all the same as eating crayons! Flavonoids protect plants from microbes, insects and fungi and so it's not surprising that they inhibit bacteria and viruses in humans. They are also known to help modify certain cell responses, thus boosting health, and additionally acting in ways that are anti-allergic or anti-cancer. Some flavonoids you may have heard of include *catechins*, which are found in green tea, and *quercetin,* found in apples.

Alkaloids are bitter tasting, nitrogen containing compounds with a wide range of effects, sometimes health promoting and sometimes damaging. Two specific examples are caffeine and morphine.

Carotenoids are also plant pigments that are known to aid the immune system in addition to having many other positive effects on the body. Lycopene is a carotenoid (tomatoes, watermelon, pink grapefruit) associated with prostate health as well as with its potential for preventing breast cancer.

Now it makes more sense why you'd want to fill your plate with colorful fruits and vegetables — these colorful pigments promote good health. And bear in mind that we discover more about plant secondary metabolites and their beneficial health effects every year.

Every so often people come up with a pill or drink that they claim contains all the nutrients necessary for life. They put all the "latest discoveries" inside that pill or drink and tell us that with this magic, we no longer need to go to the trouble of buying, cooking or storing food. But there's so much we don't know. Take tomatoes for instance. Tomatoes are recently celebrated for containing lycopene, a carotenoid associated with reduced cancer risk. Tomatoes are packed with vitamins, minerals and other phytonutrients. There are thousands of chemical compounds in tomatoes that are yet to be distinguished and understood. How can we have the short-sightedness and the hubris to assume that we know enough that we can simply extract the lycopene from tomatoes and call that sufficient?

We know that whole food sources contain many nutrients we know little about and many more that we haven't yet identified. We are discovering that nutrients generally work synergistically, meaning that certain plant constituents work better together than in isolation. For that reason and more, it makes so much more sense to eat the whole foods rather than rely on extracts of even a hundred different vitamins, minerals or nutrients.

> ***Free Radicals*** *are molecules that are highly reactive because they have an unpaired or "free" electron. These reactions damage cells and may further activate an inflammatory response. Free radicals can be useful in attacking foreign substances, but you don't want them hanging around your healthy cells. Antioxidants neutralize free radicals.*

Sure, it's more trouble to prepare whole foods for your diet. So is being sick.

Antioxidants Yes, Counting Calories, No

You've probably heard that particular foods are high in something called antioxidants, or that they are anti-inflammatory. These qualities go with various chemical compounds in plants. They can be associated with either primary or secondary metabolites.

For example, a primary metabolite (a fat) that is highly anti-inflammatory is the essential omega-3 fatty acid.

A secondary metabolite that has anti-inflammatory action is resveratrol which is found in red grapes, blueberries, chocolate and even peanut butter.

Beneficial actions, like the ability to decrease inflammation or reverse oxidation, are not unique to any single compound, nor are they only found in secondary metabolites[p]. A flavonoid like quercetin can have multiple chemical actions that include being anti-inflammatory, anti-allergic (it blocks histamine), antioxidant, anti-cancer (it regulates cell cycles and inhibits tumor growth) and anti-viral. But beta-carotene, a compound from the carotenoid family of secondary metabolites, can also do these things. It's also important to realize that just because quercetin and beta-carotene have some of the same effects, we cannot expect them to substitute for each other in the diet. We benefit from both —

---

[p] For example, selenium and zinc, minerals found in meat, act as antioxidants.

from a whole host of various antioxidants, anti-inflammatories, etc. This is one reason it's important to eat a variety of fruits and vegetables — so we can have a full arsenal of beneficial compounds.

Good eating is nutritionally dense, and it's not about how many calories you've downed. All calories are *not* created equal. There are multiple paths in your unique body that contribute to how your body handles foods. So if you and your girlfriend share a pizza, your body will handle that pizza differently in some ways from how your neighbor's body will handle the pizza she ate.

Not only do you burn calories differently from the person next to you, but you undoubtedly know that calories from one carbohydrate source are not equivalent to those of another source in terms of nutrient content.

Anti-oxidants

Highly reactive, oxygen easily reacts with other chemicals and creates FREE RADICALS.

Free radicals attack healthy cells in their attempts to stabilize themselves. Anti-oxidants can stabilize free radicals before they attack healthy cells.

Anti-oxidants are found in foods and trace minerals.

Some foods that are high in anti-oxidants include: beans (red, black, pinto, kidney), blueberries (wild ones have 1.5 times as much as cultivated), cranberries, artichoke hearts, blackberries, prunes, strawberries, apples, pecans, plums, cherries, russet potatoes.

Animal crackers or pancakes won't give you the same nutrients as plantains or parsnips. Nine grams of coconut oil won't benefit your body the same way nine grams of another fat source might, or the same way coconut oil might benefit your best friend. Foods are unique and they uniquely affect your body.

Eating a nutrient dense diet requires more than a wink and a nod to fruits and vegetables. The average American hardly eats fruits and vegetables, and some think of a side salad as a sufficient vegetable serving for the day. Compared to higher calorie sugary foods (almost any processed foods qualify) fruits and vegetables are much bulkier and far lower in calories. So fruits and vegetables will physically fill you up and provide significantly more nutrition, yet be far lower in calories than your average TV dinner.

Why don't we eat far more fruits and vegetables? Unfortunately, many of us don't enjoy the taste of vegetables and fruits. I think that instead of letting ourselves experience a wide variety of tastes, we have instead, probably inadvertently, limited ourselves to eating only what we believe tastes good. But our taste buds have been hijacked.

Who Hijacked My Taste Buds?

Our taste buds are designed to respond strongly to sugars and fats. Commercial food companies know this, and as a result they have identified something they called the "bliss" point. The bliss point is essentially the amount of sugar, fat and salt required to make a person want to eat more of that particular food.

Sugars are not nearly as common in nature as they are in our grocery. The average American eats a tremendous amount of sugar each year. Of the 150-plus pounds of added sugar the average American eats each year, only about 30 pounds are added to food by the person actually eating it. The rest has been added by the food industry. Some of the sugar included in this statistic goes into pet food[q], so it doesn't really count in processed food you or I would eat. But even so, if you compare our 150 pounds or even 30 pounds per year to the 2 pounds or so of sugar that the average American ate per year 200 years ago, you can see that we have a big sugar problem.[r]

Our taste buds and brains work to help us identify sugar and want it, because sweetness used to be (back in our hunter-gathering days) a reliable indicator of good nutrition. Blueberries are sweet and incredibly healthy, for example. But many commercially processed foods have been specifically designed to be "hyperpalatable."

Hyperpalatable foods are foods designed to contain large amounts of sugars, salts and fats that actually overwhelm the brain and stimulate the same parts of our brain that respond to heroin and cocaine.

After consuming too many of these hyperpalatable foods, our brains start to show impaired functioning, causing us to want more and more, even when we struggle to tell ourselves to stop eating.

---

[q]What?! Pets foods need added sugar?

[r] Houston? Houston?

It can take many weeks of persistent healthy eating to re-set our brains so that they are reliable guides to true hunger again.

A Vegetable & Fruit-Based Diet Contains Plenty of Protein

Lots of people worry incessantly about getting enough protein on a vegetarian or vegan diet. If so, they might be stuck again in Magic Bullet thinking. Dietary success is not a simple chemistry experiment where you add just the right amount of five different substances and presto— you have achieved health!

Just like depression is not about a "chemical imbalance" (yeah, really, it's not and we've known that for a long, long time), health and appropriate weight aren't simply about eating less food or downing more protein. If it were, a million more Americans would be at normal weights, because millions of Americans are really striving to lose excess weight by eating less and/or consuming larger amounts of protein. People generally don't get discouraged about losing weight because they just can't hack giving up the extra-large sodas or the second helpings, but because eating less food, or low-fat food hasn't worked for them. It's time to try eating differently.

So let's talk about vegetables and protein.

Proteins are crucial — they build tissue, enzymes, hormones, antibodies and even DNA. But protein consumption can be a controversial subject, and there are many impassioned arguers who take sides on issues such as animal vs. vegetable proteins, lots of protein vs. just enough,

> ### *Food and Mood:*
> ### *More Connections*
>
> *Lack of protein can make you feel unmotivated.*
>
> *When your stomach doesn't have enough acidity to digest protein, you may become protein malnourished even if you eat enough protein. You're also more vulnerable to pathogens, you may have heartburn, be constipated or develop leaky gut.*
>
> *Your body's resultant lack of protein is stressful and results in increased cortisol, which in turn raises blood sugar and affects your emotions.*
>
> *Chronically raised cortisol and elevated blood glucose further impact the body, depleting adrenals, resulting in exhaustion and even more emotional upset. Vulnerability to disease increases.*
>
> *To improve digestion:*
> *1) Don't eat while stressed: Your ability to produce stomach acids is limited when you are stressed. Chew your food: saliva contains enzymes that help digestion.*
> *2) Don't dilute stomach acid by hydrating just before a meal.*

or even when to use protein in order to gain the most muscle.

Remember the nine essential amino acids? The kinds of, and amounts of each of the essential amino acids in a food are what authorities use to determine whether that particular food is a "good" source of protein.

Hence, the term "complete" protein. A complete protein is a food that contains sufficient amounts of each of the essential amino acids, as recommended by authorities like the Institute of Medicine or the USDA.

In the last chapter we talked about how scientists interpret data based on their assumptions about the world. Guidelines for how much total protein we need and how much we need of each of the essential amino acids are also based on interpretation of empirical evidence. Here again you will see that the data we rely on is not unbiased data: it has already been made into a story.

In the 1950's a researcher named William Rose determined how much of each of the essential amino acids was needed for an average person. He took the data from the person in his study who required the highest amount of amino acids, then doubled that number and called that doubled number the minimum recommended daily intake. He felt that this doubling would insure that every body type got enough protein. His numbers are actually what have formed much of the basis for today's government recommendations for protein requirements.

You might think that this kind of approach to protein guidelines would result in an overconsumption of protein by nearly all of us, but here's where the empirical method gets even more sticky. Since we are limited by our methods, we cannot measure what we don't know to measure, and our methods of measurement limit our results. Over thirty years after Rose's experiment, amino acids were again examined using a different methodology,[24] and it was concluded that, if anything, the previous requirements erred in being too low. But on the other hand, evidence from yet another source (the book *The China Study)* that examined health outcomes of thousands of people indicated that our current USDA recommended protein requirements are actually far too high, not too low. To reiterate, it's hard to lean on empirical evidence alone to identify the truth. Data is always interpreted in a context, and that context influences the final story.

If we look more closely at some things we are pretty sure of about food, we may find some direction on this protein question. Plants provide all the nutrients we need (the primary metabolites of fat, protein, carbohydrates, vitamins and minerals) if we eat enough of them. Plants also provide thousands of beneficial secondary metabo-lites, or phytochemicals. Meat is an excellent source of protein and of some vitamins and minerals but contains no phytochemicals or fiber. Meat is also inflammatory. There is a lot of controversy regarding whether or not meat is easier to digest or harder to digest than plants. One factor playing into the controversy here is how much hydrochloric acid (HCL) is produced in each individual's stomach, as this can vary from person to person and plays a huge role in digestion. Finally, we can consider Mother Nature's provisions for protein content! Interestingly, human breastmilk is about 5%

> **Some Plants that are Complete Proteins:**
>
> Quinoa
> Amaranth
> Buckwheat
> Hemp seeds
> Chia seeds

protein, yet most authorities (like the Institute of Medicine or the USDA) recommend that adults consume a higher percentage of protein in their diets than infants apparently require. I've seen recommendations for dietary protein that range from 8% to 17% of the total diet for the average adult. Given that infants are growing at a rate that requires more protein than perhaps at any other time in their lives, the 5% amount in breastmilk leads me to question whether or not we ever need a bigger percentage of protein than we did in infancy.

Myths About Protein

Perhaps two of the most common myths about protein are these ideas: 1) meat is the only good quality protein out there, and 2) vegetables are inferior and incomplete sources of protein.

In fact, many people are surprised to learn that vegetables contain any protein (or fat) at all. Vegetables can indeed be high quality sources of complete protein if you use them in these ways: Eat a variety of vegetables so you ingest all the essential amino acids. Some vegetables don't contain all of them, and most vegetables don't have enough of each of them to be considered a complete protein. Identify the vegetables, seeds or grains that are complete proteins, and incorporate them into your diet as much as you can.

Certainly if you are only eating one or two lettuce leaves and a couple cherry tomatoes, you won't be getting any sort of adequate protein from vegetables.[s] You have to eat lots of fruits and vegetables, and treat them as your primary source of food. When people consider meat to be a "superior" source of protein, the only reason for this is that small amounts of meat contain quite a bit of protein in terms of total grams. Vegetables contain fewer total grams of protein per serving, but by percentage of protein per calorie, vegetables contain more protein than you might think! For example, ground beef is about 40% protein by calories, and cucumbers are about 20% protein by calories. However, cucumbers are also significantly lower in calories and much higher in nutritional value. Since meat is more calorically dense than are vegetables and fruit, you'll ingest far more unnecessary calories when you obtain protein from meat instead of vegetables.

More is not always better. In the case of protein, numerous studies have demonstrated that animal protein is more problematic for the body than vegetable proteins. For a more complete discussion of this issue, refer to Dr. Joel Fuhrman's excellent book, *Eat to Live.*

Low Fat, Low Help

One common misconception is that eating low-fat foods is necessary to any healthy diet. Some of you may have heard the argument that given the amount of weight gain Americans have experienced over the past 30 years and the

---

[s] Fun facts: Watermelon contains three times as much protein as an apple. The inner leaf of a head of romaine lettuce has a different amino acid profile than the outer leaf.

---

concurrent emphasis on low-fat food over those same decades, the low fat food must not be doing the trick. I agree with this conclusion: Eating low-fat food isn't the goal.

Certainly eating a lot of fat can be a potential problem, but really it depends more on what kind of fat. Likewise, not eating enough fat is a health problem. In our Magic Bullet thinking we have indiscriminately lumped fat into the "bad" category.

Fats are critical for the body to function properly. For example, myelin, the fatty sheath that enables brain cells to communicate, is made of fats. Fat is also necessary to protect organs, and it helps manage hormones. Without enough fat, the brain cannot function.

The body needs a number of different kinds of fat, but can't produce all of them on its own. The body therefore has a preference for consuming fat. As long as you use your rational brain to make good choices, this fact of nature is a good thing. A creamy avocado is packed with nutrition and your body finds it delicious. Smell and texture are part of what create this allure. In fact, taste buds can discriminate fat content in foods, and there are brain cells entirely dedicated to responding to the texture of fat. But beyond this, your saliva contains an enzyme called lingual lipase that will break down fats in your mouth within 1 to 5 seconds.[25] Interestingly, it's possible that this quick breakdown is the largest factor in what makes fat appealing to our taste buds. When rats were given fats plus a lingual lipase inhibitor that stopped them from quickly breaking down the fats into free fatty acids, the rats quickly stopped having a preference for fatty foods. [26] So it seems that enzyme breakdown plays a role in our taste preferences. This matter of taste preference is scientifically complex![27]

One of the primary reasons people have traditionally stayed away from one great source of fat — coconut oil — was the thinking that saturated fats promote heart disease, and the fact that coconut oil is loaded with saturated fats (over 90%!). However, according to recent research it appears that dietary saturated fats are actually not related to cardiac disease.[28] Rather, their medium chain triglycerides can, in reality, be therapeutic for the brain and are metabolized differently in the body as compared to long chain triglycerides. One of the results of medium chain triglyceride fat metabolism is increased energy. And research has shown that consuming 2 tablespoons per day of coconut oil creates enough energy to actually cause fat loss rather than fat gain! Furthermore, with those two tablespoons of coconut oil in your system, over 24 hours, your energy expenditure increases by 5% (that's about 120 calories).[29] Coconut oil is also somewhat anti-bacterial, anti-fungal[t] and anti-viral. This is a consequence of its high concentration of lauric acid (about 50%). Fresh coconut oil tastes great and seems to help people eat less, particularly if you have it with breakfast. Coconut oil also helps improve blood lipids, resulting in lower LDL cholesterol, higher HDL cholesterol, and reduced triglycerides.

---

[t] It's also the best thing ever in the bedroom, if you know what I mean. The anti-fungal properties can help protect against Candida, whereas some commercially available lubricating products may encourage yeast infections due to their sugar content.

What About Plants and Fats?

We also often think of animal products as primary sources for our essential fatty acids, the omega fats. However, nutritional analysis shows that in a comparison of kale and chicken, kale is your best bet for omega fats. Kale contains 121 mg of omega-3 fatty acids compared to chicken's 98 mg. The omega story comparing animal versus plant sources becomes even more interesting when we look at omega-6 fatty acid amounts. Omega-6 fatty acids are necessary for bodily functioning, but most Americans consume far, far too many of them. Keeping a healthy ratio of omega-3's to omega-6's is key for good health (1 to 3 or 1 to 4 is a pretty good idea; most Americans have a ratio of 1 to 20 or thereabouts). Kale contains just 92 mg of omega-6 fatty acid, for a ratio of 1 to less than 1, while chicken contains 826 mg, making the ratio of omega-3's to omega-6's in chicken about 1 to 8.5. This is about the same ratio found in homemade whole wheat bread (146 mg omega-3's to 1206 omega-6's), so if you are having a chicken sandwich on your favorite aunt's hearty whole wheat bread, you'll want to add quite a lot of kale to that sandwich in order to improve the ratio of omega-3's to omega-6's.

But I don't want to give up my food pleasure!

Along the road to eating more plant based foods, there can be another sticking point for many people who may believe that it's not possible to experience culinary pleasure, – real, honest to goodness pleasure – in eating plants. I've tasted the average supermarket vegetable and believe me, I really hear you. If I were a conspiracy theorist, I'd think fast food companies were in charge of selling us supermarket vegetables so we'd forget what real food tastes like.

We drown vegetables in sugar, salt and fats because they don't taste good enough to us. But it's not because they *can't* taste good. Perhaps the poor vegetables are just not that fresh[u], because fresh, well-grown vegetables taste wonderful! It's all the sugar, salt and fat we've been eating for years that has derailed our body's natural appetite chemistry so that our taste buds don't work like they should. What this means is this: we may be unable to taste how good vegetables actually are because we have limited our taste buds through our own eating history.

The solution to that is to retrain the brain so that it can experience "real food!" You may not like the most highly nutritious foods on the planet at first, but that doesn't mean you can't learn to love them. Your taste buds can and will change if you give them enough opportunity. We'll talk more about this later in the book.

Emotions and Food

Overeating is a problem that affects us mentally, emotionally and physically. It can feel very discouraging to be a habitual overeater! There are plenty of reasons to look at what compels us to overeat, resulting in increased blood sugar, fat and poorer sleep. One primary

---

[u] Sometimes it's a long journey from South America.

reason we overeat is that we are eating out of unmet emotional needs, not out of hunger.

Emotions often drive choices that we might not make when we're not "under the influence" of those emotions. When a person experiences emotions, it's a whole body thing. Emotions have a physiological impact in your body. Neurotransmitters (chemical messengers that "send" thoughts around your brain), and hormones that affect heart rate and blood sugar are not imaginary but real physiological events. So emotions leave a physical trace. The body has to clean this up, just like everything else. The body does this by metabolizing, excreting, and breaking down the physiological hormone detritus left by our emotions. Your liver helps in this process. But if the liver is way too busy helping you clean up after last night's cheesecake or bout of drinking, then it isn't as available to break down emotional byproducts. Priorities are priorities, and alcohol will trump leftover hormones on the clean-up list.

There is a growing body of research that explores how various plants, including both traditional foods and medicinal herbs, can assist the body in these kinds of healing tasks. For instance, dandelions are pretty well known for their powerful healing effects on the liver. Not only that, dandelions are also high in calcium and iron, have more protein than spinach (14%), are packed with vitamins and minerals and have anti-inflammatory effects.

Just don't eat the ones that have been sprayed with herbicides and pesticides.

Since we hear so much about healing plants from the Asian side of the globe, it may appear that the folks in India and China have incredibly powerful medicinal plants growing practically on top of each other. But it's not that there are fewer medicinal plants in the Americas. Instead, there is a tremendous bias in the research on the subject. Lots of research into medicinal plants has been funded in Asia, and much less money has been spent on similar research here in the United States. Not only that, the long standing tradition of herbal medicine in Asian cultures has been left far more intact than here in America where that culture was noisily stamped out to prevent competition with conventional medicine.

Not only can increasing your vegetable intake assist you in your quest for mind-body health, but herbs can be valuable adjuncts to healing. Be careful, however, that you don't place too much confidence in the ability of herbal medicine to make up for eating poorly in the first place. Herbs can help the body in many different ways and when consumed with wisdom and prudence they can be extremely useful. But if we are ignoring the basics of health (that three-legged stool of dietary intake, sleep and exercise) we cannot fix our problems by simply taking a

> *If we are ignoring the basics of health we cannot fix the problems by simply taking a bunch of medicinal plants. If you're eating hot dogs and drinking soda there's no way herbal preparations are powerful enough to fix that. It's like a tidal wave versus a current.*

bunch of medicinal plants (just like pharmaceutical meds cannot fix habit problems very effectively – you have to actually change your life). If you're eating hot dogs and drinking soda there's no way herbal preparations are powerful enough to fix that. It's like a tidal wave versus a current.

When you are eating nutritionally dense meals, you are less likely to engage in emotional eating. You feel good because your body and brain are receiving the nutrition they need to function optimally. You are happier and more resilient, and you will simply find that there are far fewer good reasons to grab a donut.

Eating nutritionally dense meals is one of the legs on our three-legged stool. The next two chapters discuss the other two legs of that stool: sleep and exercise.

Chapter Seven

Sleep

Tasha wandered hazily into my office and flopped into her chair. She looked unhappy, so down in fact that I was instantly worried that something really bad had happened.

"Are you okay?" I asked, a note of concern in my voice.

"Meh," she replied, not even half-heartedly. "I guess."

"Did something happen?" I was not at all comforted by her weak answer.

"Oh, not really. No..."

Tasha is fifteen and isn't trying to be difficult. She's mostly just fifteen. The obsessive-compulsive disorder she struggles with makes it hard for her to manage homework and school. She landed in my office because of OCD, but it looks to me that OCD is a secondary problem. Because she tends to be anxiety-prone, lack of sleep, exercise and poor nutrition make life all the more difficult for her. She has a particularly hard time accepting that she really does need to get to bed earlier.

Since my previous queries had yielded no result, I ventured down a different track.

"Boy, then, you sure sound blah. Not enough sleep last night?"

I gave her a sort of conspiratorial smile, encouraging her to be up front with her answer. She knows that I really get it – what fifteen year-old wants to go to bed at 10 when her friends are still texting?

"No. I couldn't fall asleep," she groaned. "And then I had a really bad morning because I was so tired."

Mornings have a way of not cooperating when you've had a bad night, don't they? That's pretty much a given. And with this client (and most clients – and most of you!), before we can work on the OCD or any other problem, we have to straighten out the sleep.

Not only is it significantly more difficult to work on any of life's problems when you're not getting enough sleep, it's also harder to tolerate ups and downs of any kind. You just have very little resilience. All that extra emotional turbulence makes it hard to solve problems, and I have often found that once the sleep is straightened out, remaining symptoms are distinctly less severe and sometimes hardly present at all.

Circadian Rhythm and Sleep

We sleep based on a circadian rhythm, the "master clock" of the body. Circadian rhythm on the inside is connected to the circadian rhythm of outside light and dark cycles controlled by the spinning earth, sun and moon.

Yes, the moon affects our sleep[30]. In a study done over a three year time span, researchers had participants sleep in a sleep lab where there was no exposure to the sky (and therefore no moonlight). Data showed that during the three to four nights surrounding the full moon, participants fell asleep about five minutes later than usual and that their overall sleep was about 20 minutes shorter than usual, on average. There were also brain and chemical changes: brain waves that indicate deep sleep were 30% less frequent than on non-full moon nights, and melatonin levels were also lower.

Though the moon can influence our sleep rhythm to a mild extent, it's the daily rising of the sun that influences us most. One of the benefits of (and perhaps a reason for) an internal circadian rhythm is that it influences our body organs so that they can work together on a schedule that allows them maximum efficiency without interfering with each other.

We used to think that it was just the brain that had a circadian rhythm, but we now understand that every organ in our body has its own clock, and functions accordingly. For example, if the liver and pancreas are out of sync, insulin production will suffer. And since our bodies are tied to the sun in terms of their primary source for a circadian rhythm, sleep that is out of sync with the sun will also be out of sync with what our bodies need. Sleep is not just a time for rest. It's a time when lots of things happen in your body — things that won't get to happen if you are awake.

Let me put it another way: our bodies were not designed to work all night and sleep all day, or stay up dancing until one in the morning. There's a price to pay for sleep deprivation. It involves much more than our merely being tired or needing caffeine to get going the next morning. The price involves our whole body and our health.[v]

Our internal clock operates on a cellular level. That clock will keep time even when we are stuck in the dark for long periods (this ability to keep time despite lack of day-night light differences is called "free-running"). Light resets our clocks each day and begins a marvelous cascade of chemical, hormonal changes throughout the body.

In the morning, light signals the body to stop production of melatonin. Melatonin is a hormone that does a number of things throughout the body but is best known for its role in sleep. Melatonin is produced according to the body's circadian rhythm. There is a natural cycle that causes melatonin to rise throughout the evening before bedtime and then fall to low levels in the morning. Melatonin is also a powerful antioxidant and plays a big role in regulating the immune system, moods, reproductive systems

---

[v] Although, if you are in generally good health, you'll pay a lower price than a person who is in generally poorer health.

and even in helping combat certain viral and bacterial infections.

Just goes to show that we can't simplify anything! Melatonin is usually thought of as the sleep helper, but it is such a powerful healer that it has created startling recoveries in infants with sepsis[31], been shown to treat migraines, reduces the severity and incidence of gastric ulcers, and is known as one of the most powerful scavengers of free radicals.[32]

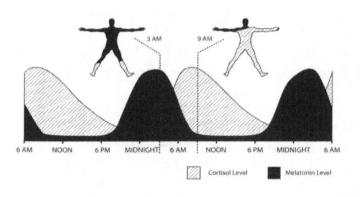

Morning light also signals the body clock to start production of serotonin, adrenalin and cortisol. A surge in cortisol is what pulls us out of deep sleep, but the relatively higher levels of cortisol in the morning are only meant to stay in your body for a short time, just enough to get you up and going.

Cortisol levels, like melatonin, are also cyclical, and rise or fall depending on the time of day. As melatonin levels are rising in the evening, cortisol levels are dropping off so that you can relax and go to sleep. While cortisol levels drop throughout the day, adrenalin and serotonin levels continue to increase, ramping up the metabolism. Body temperature rises and we increase in activity and then appetite as the liver and stomach become ready to process nutrients.

Your metabolism is at peak by the mid-afternoon, which is a great time to exercise, as the body is most efficient at turning fat into energy at this time. For the same reason, mid-afternoon is also a better time to eat your heaviest meal.

By evening, the light is fading, and consequently production of the activating hormones also fades. Body temperature decreases and some of that serotonin begins to be converted into melatonin. This onset of increased melatonin levels is called Dim Light Melatonin Onset (DLMO). DLMO timing varies for people, depending on their own circadian rhythm, but it is heavily dependent on dimmed lights. If you are living in bright light until 10 pm or later, it's very likely that your DLMO just won't work well, and your sleep cycle won't line up with daylight and nighttime, creating potential problems.

By the way, when melatonin is higher, your body moves a bit toward a semi-hibernation state in which it becomes more efficient at holding onto carbs and fat and converting them into storage instead of burning them. So you want to eat your high carb and high fat meals at lunchtime, and at least four hours before bedtime (and we're talking about a regular bedtime, not an extra-late midnight bedtime).

What happens about two hours after DLMO (Dim Light Melatonin Onset) is that your body becomes flooded with melatonin. Melatonin isn't quite at its nighttime peak in terms of how high the level is, but it is circulating faster through the body at this time than any other time during the rest of the night. This is the best time to fall asleep. Within an hour, the release of melatonin will slow down and it will become more difficult to fall asleep.

Sometimes people stay awake and then get a second wind or feel less sleepy. In part, this is because they have missed that prime window of opportunity when melatonin was flowing faster. Also, you can stimulate the production of more cortisol by refusing to go to sleep when your body tells you it's tired. Years of ignoring sleep signals in your body can teach you to be relatively unaware that you are tired. And, not only can the kind of foods you eat keep you awake longer than helpful but you might also eat so late in the evening that you remain awake past the DLMO induced window.

Sleep Opportunity and Light

Remember well that this window of sleep opportunity is tied to light. It's not tied to your TV schedule, or to what most of society considers to be normative at night. It's probably significantly earlier than you think it "should" be. I certainly know for myself that there have been many times when I've refused to go to bed because I've thought it was too early. If I choose to force myself to stay awake, I become subjectively less tired as the minutes tick by, and eventually I have trouble falling asleep at what I'd like to be the "right" time.

So if you dim the lights in your home around eight p.m., figuring that's close to DLMO for you, you'll find it easier to fall asleep at ten p.m.

Think that's too early? In one study, adults were not given any toys to play with before bed (things like computers, TV, etc.), and additionally were not given any clues as to what time it was. After a few very boring evenings, their sleep schedules changed and they ended up falling asleep regularly around nine p.m. In the absence of distractions, your body will tell you what time to go to bed. You'll feel better if you listen.

Shift Work

One more thing about the power of light over bedtime: Sometimes people do choose to shift their sleep schedules. Exposure to bright light can do this when applied before bedtime, or upon wakening. If you allow yourself to be in bright light before bed, you'll fall asleep later, and you'll wake up later. The later in the evening you are exposed to this bright light, the longer you will be delayed in falling asleep. But about five hours after your usual bedtime (if your bedtime is usually at eleven p.m., this would be around four a.m.), your body temperature hits its lowest point. When your body is at this low temperature point, any bright light exposure from then until daybreak will cause you to wake up earlier and fall asleep sooner at the end of the day. Bright light does this effectively until about two hours after your regular wakeup time, at which point bright light has pretty much no effect on your sleep and wake cycle. That's because your body is trained to be in bright light during the day.[w]

Melatonin is continuously released throughout the night until the body perceives a gradual light increase, which the body can do through the eyelids. As darkness fades, so does melatonin production (usually about 1-2 hours before awakening)

There are cells in your eyes called ipRGC's (intrinsically photosensitive retinal ganglion cells) that control how light affects your circadian rhythms. The ipRGC cells respond most powerfully to blue light. Think about what color the sky is at dawn. Blue, right? How about that. These cells send signals to the pineal gland in the brain, informing it about how light it is outside.

Ever wake up and stand at the window, looking out at the dawn? And you sometimes just suddenly feel awake? This may be the melatonin in your system getting an abrupt shutdown from your exposure to light. Light can significantly reduce melatonin, and that's why light can create such problems at night. Blue-lit screens like those on phones, computers and TVs can wreak havoc on your circadian rhythms. They will send you the "it's dawn!" signal even though it's 10:30 at night, and you will, as a result, become less sleepy.

---

[w] Yes, I'm being Dr. Obvious here. Glad you caught that.

Sleep Deprivation

Did you know that if you deprive a fruit fly of sleep, it experiences cognitive impairment (as measured by things like how long it takes the fly to learn where the sugar is, and how quickly the fly forgets)?[33] Even fruit flies with their very little brains need their beauty rest.[x]

We know that sleep is crucial to our health, but we probably underestimate how important it is. We think we can get away with 6 or 7 hours per night because we think that amount is so close to what we need that it shouldn't matter. After all, the only symptom we seem to feel is a little bit of tiredness, and after we get up in the morning (and drink caffeine) that quickly fades.

Average Sleep Needs (according to NIH)

Age	Hours
Newborns (0-2 months)	12 – 18
Infants (3 months to 1 year)	14 – 15
Toddlers (1 to 3 years)	12 – 14
Preschoolers (3 to 5 years)	11 – 13
School-aged (5 to 12 years)	10 – 11
Teens (12 to 18 years)	8.5 – 10
Adults (18+)	7.5 - 9

America is actually full of people with chronic sleep deprivation. A common myth about

---

[x] Interesting note: birds can sleep with one brain hemisphere at a time, while the other hemisphere stays awake and alert. Dolphins and seals do this too.

sleep is that getting just an hour less than normal per night won't affect you. We've heard that we need about eight hours of sleep; however, most people think of those 8 hours as a luxury, unrealistic in their current life. Some people even think of an eight hour night's sleep as near to indolence, much less as actually healthy. But the fact is that getting even one hour less sleep per night will affect your ability to think properly and respond quickly to problems. It also compromises your cardiovascular health, your balance of energy and your immune system's ability to fight infection.[34]

We may think we can adapt to simply sleeping less, but what we are adapting to instead is how tired we are. We become quite good at not knowing, or noticing our fatigue. We may get used to not sleeping enough for months or even years, and all this time, continue to believe that we are doing okay. But then we are surprised when accidents happen because our subjective judgment all along was simply that we weren't *that* tired.

You cannot adapt to getting less sleep than you require. You may think you can, but you are just not aware of how impaired you are. Your brain literally remembers how long you've been asleep and awake and keeps track of this for weeks, and "...the bigger our aggregate sleep deficit, the faster our performance deteriorates, even after a good night's rest."[35] Chronic sleep loss means that even when you have a good long night's sleep, you will still tire much faster than you would if you weren't under a sleep debt.

Another reason people think they are less tired than they actually are (other than, of

---

The Sleep Cycle

Stage One: Relaxation. *This stage only lasts 5-10 minutes. You're probably unaware you are asleep. The brain gives off beta waves that gradually become alpha waves. Alpha brainwaves are associated with meditating or daydreaming.*
Stage Two: Light sleep. *The brain gives off theta waves, brainwaves also associated with meditation.*
Stage Three: Deep Sleep. *Non-dreaming, restorative sleep. The brain gives off delta waves.*
Stage Four: Deepest Sleep. *Just like stage three, only deeper. The brain continues delta waves.*
REM sleep: *Rapid Eye Movement sleep in which we dream. Brainwaves resemble wakefulness. The first REM cycle occurs about 90 minutes after we fall asleep and lasts only about ten minutes. The final REM cycle of the night can last about an hour.*

---

course, our natural tendency to assume we are right and we know everything) is that we tend to judge how tired we are based on how we feel between 3 and 7 pm. Since we are hitting the high point of our circadian cycle at that time of day, we naturally feel better. That's because melatonin levels are at their lowest, and this phenomenon essentially masks the effects of sleep loss.

To make matters worse, the bigger our sleep debt, the less capable we are of understanding that we have a big sleep debt. Most of us can hardly remember what it's like to feel fully rested, so we start to believe that we are more fully rested than we actually are.

The National Sleep Foundation (NSF) reports that at least 40 million Americans have a sleep disorder, and that 60% of Americans report sleep problems at least a few nights per week. The numbers are worse for children – nearly 70% experience sleep problems at least a few nights per week.

We often think that older people need less sleep, but this is yet another myth that simply isn't true. Older people often get less sleep, but they still need just as much sleep as they did earlier in their lives. The ability to slide into deep, restful sleep stages decreases with age. A more fragile sleeper is more easily disturbed by things like noise, light, pain and any special medical problems that may also contribute to sleep difficulties.

Sleep and Learning

We've known for a long time that sleep improves learning. I remember hearing about studies decades ago that examined the impact of sleep sessions between learning sessions. Essentially sleep was shown to help consolidate learning, and sleep was found to be more helpful between study sessions than any other activity, including more studying!

What we may not realize is that not only is sleep helpful, it's truly necessary to good learning. Without enough sleep we can't remember things we have learned before or after that sleep period.

So if you pull an all-nighter, you won't keep much of that information in your long-term memory, even if you do pass the test. [36]

How Do You Know You're Sleepy?

Signs of sleepiness can include more than yawning or just feeling tired. Most people know that it's common to be irritable and moody when they are sleepy, but disinhibition (losing good judgment) is also one of the first signs a person will show when sleepy.

Yes, being sleepy is a lot like being impaired by alcohol.

If you still insist on remaining awake despite those signs, you might begin feeling apathetic, like you just don't care about things that you used to care about. Your emotional reactivity "flattens," meaning that you don't have the usual vividness to your emotional responses. Your speech can slow down, you'll forget things, creativity is a problem and it becomes really hard to do more than one thing at once.

When the fatigue gets quite bad, you start having microsleeps, small periods of sleeping that last for 5-10 seconds. This can happen while driving, listening, reading, etc. Grimly enough, what comes next – if you don't simply fall asleep – is hallucinations.

The similarity to alcohol abuse is sobering, isn't it?[y]

---

[y] I couldn't help myself.

An Expert Speaks

"I have treated sleep disorders in children for many years, having been trained by an internationally-famous authority in that area. I have treated a TON of kids. What I can tell you (and this is borne out by the research) is that when a child is diagnosed with Attention Deficit / Hyperactivity Disorder (ADHD) there is almost always a significant sleep problem. In the past this link has been assumed to mean that the ADHD causes the sleep disorder, but in fact it may well be the other way around. I found that once I corrected the sleep problems, the so-called ADHD problems just went away. See, rather than getting drowsy, kids try to over-compensate when they feel tired, and become (as one expert put it) "tired and wired." Very often, this "tired and wired" presentation is assumed to be ADHD, when in fact it is sleep deprivation. One study had kids go to bed an hour earlier than usual and another group of kids go to bed an hour later than usual. Guess what? Those who went to bed an hour later than usual had what might be considered ADHD symptoms.

Dr. Mack Stephenson, Boise, Idaho

And there actually is a relationship between alcohol abuse and poor sleep. Teen boys who had poor *preschool* sleep habits were twice as likely to use drugs and alcohol and tobacco as compared to teens with healthy preschool sleep habits, even when researchers controlled this study for issues like depression, aggression, attention problems and parental alcoholism. We're talking about the consequences of sleep patterns your parents helped create for you when you were three and four years old! We know there's a relationship between poor sleep and alcohol abuse in adults, but for some reason that seems less surprising than the sleep-drug connection between toddlers and teens.

Child & Adolescent Sleep

Fortunately there are some great books to help you parents help your children learn to sleep well[z]. Whatever method you choose, just remember that when it's nighttime, your child's need for sleep outweighs his or her need for anything else.

Including "love."

If you want a child with a happier, healthier and literally *smarter* brain, help them get more sleep. Young children who get even one more hour of sleep per day score significantly higher on tests of intelligence.

It's not just the preschool years that you have to focus on when it comes to sleep. Adolescence is famously problematic. We can all think of an adolescent we know of who stays up way too late, and seems to sleep all weekend.

Adolescence and Risk

Adolescence is a high risk time for developing health problems and particularly mental health problems. At least 50% of all adult mental health disorders start in adolescence, the most common among them being mood disorders

---

[z] Marc Weissbluth: *Healthy Sleep Habits, Happy Child*; Richard Ferber: *Solve Your Child's Sleep Problems*; Jody Mindell: *Sleeping Through The Night*

like anxiety, depression[aa] and bipolar disorder. Adolescents are not only faced with a multiplicity of changes in their social, developmental, academic and vocational lives, but they are faced with a biologically-driven sleep pattern that urges them to both stay up later and sleep later in the day as their circadian rhythm changes, making it much more difficult for them to go to sleep "on time" and to wake up "on time".

This physiological change happens at the same time adolescents want increased levels of independence. Although it is difficult to help adolescents see the wisdom in sleeping well and in good nutrition, it is so worth it. Poor sleep and poor nutrition combined act synergistically to create many more problems than either would separately.

It's also tough to get youth to believe you that sleep and good nutrition are important. This happens, in part, because they don't detect the differences that good vs. poor sleep and good vs. poor nutrition create in their young bodies as strongly as they will later in life.

So it's crucial to teach your kids about the importance of eating right, sleeping well and exercising regularly while they are quite young. Do them this great kindness. Emotional and behavioral regulation are hard gifts for parents to learn to give, but they pay off.

[aa] Some data report that about 73% of youth with depression also have sleeping problems. As we'll talk about in the Depression chapter later in the book, lack of sleep has been shown to be causally related to depression.

Your Brain Cycles All Night...And All Day

We're used to thinking about sleep in terms of cycles. We readily accept that our brainwaves change during sleep and that there is a natural ebb and flow to those changes as we sleep.

But during the day we assume that the brain is different. It's as though we can readily accept this lovely oscillation at night, but in the morning we think we can just flick on the switch and the brain will be on GO all day. This is not so.

In a wonderful book called *The Power of Full Engagement*, authors Jim Loehr and Tony Schwartz discuss data that indicate our brains continue their 90 minute cycles throughout the day. Of course we aren't in delta wave sleep during the day, but our brains are not simply in one phase all day long without variation. These authors' overall point is that, by taking advantage of the natural variations in our alertness, we can become more resilient and reserve more energy. As we understand and work with these 90-minute cycles during daylight hours, we will not only work better during the day but sleep better at night, in part because we are calmer overall.

Sleep Underlies Better Health

Better sleep is powerfully associated with better health. Time spent sleeping is far from wasted time, particularly as there are some bodily processes we need that only occur during sleep. Good sleep is associated with a better ability to manage digestion and less storage of fat and carbs (i.e., you can burn fat better if you sleep enough). We need good sleep to maximize the secretion of hormones like growth hormone which helps us repair our bodies and improves our metabolism. For example, recent research shows that sleep is critical for the body to be able to repair and create myelin, the protective covering for nerve cells. When people are asleep, the body produces double the number of cells that give rise to myelin than when people are awake.[37]

Sleep quality and quantity is even associated with coronary artery calcification (calcification occurs when the inner lining of an artery develops plaque, a marker for coronary heart disease). Moreover, the duration of sleep relates to things like how glucose is used and regulated in the body, blood pressure levels and weight gain and loss. All of these above variables are also related to heart disease risk factors. In a study of participants with no detectable calcification at the beginning of the study, sleep and artery calcification were measured at baseline, and then again five years later. Study participants who slept longer had significantly less calcification in their arteries[38]. The "zinger" from this study is that no other variable tracked by the researchers (gender, age, weight, etc.) had more of an impact on calcification—thanks to sleep! The take-home message here is that sleep is crucial; how much you sleep and how well you sleep are at the top of the pecking order when you consider what impacts your health.

In fact, as you realize that your sleep affects your eating habits and your exercise habits (although both of those habits in turn can affect your sleep), establishing a routine that brings you regular quality sleep can become one of your highest priorities. It will certainly make the rest of your health-related behaviors (that's everything, by the way – your feelings, your communications, how you talk to yourself, etc.!) easier to bring in line with what you intend for your life.

Fixing poor sleep is the sticky part, isn't it? Though there is a ton of advice on the internet about how to improve your sleep, I want to mention just a few things that I have found useful, both with my clients and with my own sleep, which tends to get problematic at times. Keep in mind that the following suggestions are additive – one may not do the trick by itself, but putting many of these practices together can really help you sleep better.

1. Sleep Hygiene.

a) A truly dark environment is necessary. Light lowers melatonin levels and wakes you up. Even small amounts of light make a difference, so notice your clock, the light on your phone charger, etc. Use blackout curtains if your regular curtains or shades don't entirely block sources of nighttime light. You will sleep more soundly.

b) Cooler temperatures. Your body cools off to fall asleep, so if you take a hot shower and then climb into bed in a cool room, you will fall asleep more easily. On the other hand, research shows that wearing socks to bed also improves sleep.[bb]

[bb] Not for me! I can't abide socks at night.

c) Make the bedroom about sleeping, not watching TV or doing work. Keep the bed for sleep or sex only.

d) Be sure that your pillows, blankets and mattress are comfortable. If you struggle to be comfortable, this struggle may interfere with your sleep all night long. Since people with chronic insomnia have a three times higher risk of death from any cause[39] it's totally worth it to invest in bedding that helps you sleep better.

e) You may need to use earplugs or even a separate bedroom if you have a bedmate who snores or otherwise wakes you up at night. Instead of getting irritated at your partner, take charge of your health by doing what you need to do in order to create the sleep you need.

2. A Solid Sleep Routine

a) This includes getting to bed right away when you start to feel tired. Let your sleep cycle work *for* you, not against you. Trust the system: your body gets tired automatically, and it only doesn't work when you interfere. As detailed earlier, whenever you force yourself to stay awake, you are forcing your system to adapt by finding the energy somewhere, and often this requires dumping some cortisol in your system. Then you're not sleepy and you'll stay awake much longer. Listen to your body! Catch the sleep wave the first time.

We ignore our bodies' cries for sleep, just like we ignore our children's cries for sleep. When infants get tired, they tell us. They rub their eyes or yawn. We think they are cute and wait for the clock to tell us when it's time to put them to bed.

By then they have had to dump cortisol in their little bodies to keep themselves awake for us. And then we are upset because they are running around like maniacs. Cute, isn't it?

We made it happen. We did it to them. We do it to ourselves too. So learn to listen well, and when you hear yourself getting sleepy, respond instantly.

You might prepare for bed before it's time to fall asleep so that your preparations don't wake you up. Brush your teeth before you are tired. Incidentally, peppermint oil (as opposed to peppermint leaf) can be stimulating, and is an ingredient in many toothpastes because we all seem to like that minty stimulation in our mouths. Whatever it is that you feel you need to do before bed, do it early so you aren't forced to choose between sleep and doing what you need to do before bed.

Be sure that your daytime is active. Lack of physical activity during the day leads to significantly poorer quality sleep at night. Napping during the day can erode your drive for sleep as well.

Successfully creating a solid sleep routine means that you stick to your routine all the time. You can't plan on disrupting the routine every weekend and expect it to work fine during the week. You may not like keeping such a set schedule, and that's fine. You don't have to like it or not like it. Rhythms and routines are just the way your body works! If you are unwilling to keep a set sleep schedule, you have to also be willing to pay the price, because the price will come whether or not you are ready for it. It may be poorer health, less creativity, disrupted relationships or emotional exhaustion. Keeping a solid sleep routine as a priority for several months will show you what you've been missing — and you will more easily find the time (and brainpower) to do what you want to do in the daytime!

b) Create an environment that can help bring on sleepiness. If dim light melatonin onset is part of sleepiness, make sure the environment supports that happening: for example, turn of all the overhead lights at 8 pm. Turn off the TV and the computer. Read a book with lamplight instead.

c) Do the same things in the same order every night. Teach your body through behaviors that this is the time to start moving toward sleep. Don't give up after three days. Do the same thing over and over for weeks. Your body needs to hear a lot of repetition before it starts to get it.

d) For heaven's sake, get to bed early! Don't believe you can't start thinking about bed until at least 10:30 pm. The same thing that's true for children is true for adults – if you are having trouble with sleep, try getting there earlier. Sometimes you just need more sleep in order to have better quality sleep.

Another reason to get to bed early is that your body is connected to the sun, and your circadian rhythm (including that of your internal organs) is also connected to the sun – and NOT to your late-night TV schedule. What this means is that some internal organ functioning will either happen or not happen depending on whether or not you are asleep. For example, your adrenal system does most of its rejuvenation for two hours starting about 11 pm. If you suffer from chronic exhaustion, you know your adrenal glands are suffering. If you are staying up until 11:30 or midnight, you are significantly interfering with any adrenal rest. If your gall bladder's circadian rhythm is to release toxins into the excretory system before midnight, and you are still awake, then the toxins go into your liver instead. This can create a bigger load for the liver to process when it needs to be processing other things. If it happens every night, you can imagine the problematic impact that poor, worn-out liver might have on your health.

3. Food and Drink in Relation to Sleep

When you eat large, complicated and meaty dinners, your body will have a harder time sleeping than if you eat light and simple meals at dinner. The problem becomes worse the later you eat, but even if you eat earlier, consuming a complicated meal affects your level of relaxation. Try it out for a few weeks, as I have, before you come to any conclusions.

I once ate a variety of four-item, vegetable-only (no meat, no beans, no bread, no fruit) dinners for about four weeks. For example, one dinner might have been lettuce, tomatoes, celery and carrots and as much as I wanted of only those four foods. Somewhere in the third week I experienced calmer and deeper sleep than I ever thought a four-item dinner could be responsible for. It was a real surprise. Don't knock it 'till you try it. Your digestion can keep you awake (and affect the quality of your sleep).

You know, of course, that caffeine interferes with sleep, and this includes caffeine that is consumed in the afternoon, not just at night. Take a close look at how much caffeine you are ingesting. Even decaf drinks have been shown to contain significant caffeine (amounts vary depending on where you bought that decaf coffee). But there are other stimulating foods that also interfere with sound slumber. High fat foods, foods with tyramine (which produces a stimulating hormone, norepinephrine), chocolate, sugary foods, and alcohol all interfere with sleep. Keep these to breakfast and lunch as much as you can. Cigarettes are stimulating, and interfere with sleep. Alcohol may make you feel initially sleepy, but is disruptive to sleep, as is marijuana. Both promote REM sleep which is less restful.

4. Supplements and Sleep

a) Melatonin can help, but not all melatonin is created equally. Some melatonin is of far better quality. Whether you take it in a capsule or a sublingual liquid can make a difference in how much it affects you. Also, the amount you take really matters. When I was faculty at Yale University School of Medicine, I talked to a few of the top melatonin researchers in the country. Each of them had the same thing to tell me about melatonin: the standard dosage of 3 mg is far too much. They suggested to start with about 1 mg, and further explained that smaller doses are often more effective. This is one great example where more isn't better.

When I use supplemental melatonin, I take about 0.4 to 0.7 mg. I use a sublingual, liquid melatonin that I can easily titrate to small amounts. Melatonin in this form doesn't have to be swallowed and go through the stomach before it starts working in the body. A little bit goes a long way. Another thing the experts told me was that if I felt groggy the next morning, I could try taking melatonin earlier or taking less. They assured me that I was the best person to determine how melatonin impacted my sleep and my ability to wake refreshed the next morning. You can do the same and adjust melatonin according to what your body tells you.

I don't use melatonin regularly, but when I was trying to establish a reliable sleep routine, it was very useful for a period of time. I still use it on occasion when I'm having trouble falling asleep.

b) There are a number of herbs like peppermint (leaf, not oil), valerian, passionflower, hops, etc., or herbal combinations that can be useful. But if you use them, remember there are many factors that contribute to sleep. You can't watch a shoot-em-up on TV while eating fried chicken and chocolate dipped brownies, and then expect that downing a cup of chamomile tea is going to do it.

5. Meditation and Sleep

Meditation may improve sleep on its own, but in my opinion, meditation primarily improves your ability to stop ruminating. If your primary cause of sleep trouble is that you can't let go of worries, practice regular meditation. As you learn how to get your mind to be more disciplined, your ability to manage your attention will improve, and you will be able to get yourself to stop ruminating.

Ironically, an anxious urge to get enough sleep is one of the biggest detractors from getting quality sleep. Trust your body to work for you. When you have "should" thoughts like "I should be able to fall asleep right away," or "I should be able to sleep for eight quality hours every night," let these thoughts go. Turn your mind to a meditative relaxation exercise. It's normal to have disrupted sleep every so often. Jon Kabat-Zinn has created some wonderful meditation CDs[cc] that are great tools to help you develop meditation as a pathway to increased mental discipline and peace. I highly recommend these.

To summarize, sleep is a crucial leg in our three-legged stool that supports health. Sleep is not just a switch you flip – it can be a delicate balance and routine you need to become attuned to. Respect the balance and the routine. Take time to develop the ability to nourish your whole self with the quality sleep you need in order to fully bloom as the person who you are.

[cc] www.mindfulnesstapes.com

Chapter Eight

Exercise

Y ou've probably heard of Ted Talks. I highly recommend them, not only because they are really fun to exercise to (especially if you have a nerdy love of learning random things) but also because they are so informative and entertaining.

There's a great Ted Talk by a woman named Margaret Heffernan called "The Dangers of Willful Blindness."[40] She talks about the town of Libby, Montana, and the cancer-causing vermiculite (a particularly toxic form of asbestos) that polluted the environment there as a by-product of the local mining industry. As her story goes, there was a woman who discovered, kind of by accident, the cause of the cancer that was killing so many of the people in her hometown. She tried to tell the townspeople about this problem: the vermiculite-cancer connection. Her thought was, "When everyone knows, they'll surely do something!" To her astonishment and dismay, people were surprisingly resistant, even shunning her. They were much happier to accept a 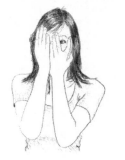 tremendously high death rate rather than the truth.

It's not just the people in that town who ignore important truths about health. We all do this thing. We Americans have a shockingly high death rate from diseases that we could fix with lifestyle changes. But all too often we do not take charge of our health destinies. We ignore our problems. We have epic willful blindness!

Exercise is prime among the crucial health practices far too many neglect.

But making exercise an integral[dd] part of your life requires change. Change is hard. (Here's where you can whine if you like. I do, sometimes!).

Yes, it's true. It's hard.

On the other hand, scientists are indeed trying to create a pill that substitutes for exercise. For real. When I was in fifth grade this would have seemed like total science fiction. My take on

---

[dd]When I was in high school, I had a goal to use the word "integral" in every single paper I wrote. It's hilarious that this very word was suggested here by an editor! Bazinga!

that endeavor: don't hold your breath. I can't imagine such a pill would come without serious adverse side effects. Don't wait to exercise because you think that one day a pill will save you.

Here's a statistic that you may find sobering. The Centers for Disease Control and Prevention found that over half of the women (60%) and half the men (50%) in the US *never* engage in any "vigorous" physical activity lasting at least ten minutes per week. Just 25% of women (31% of men) actually exercise vigorously at least ten minutes per week.[41] What an example of willful blindness!

There are all kinds of beneficial side effects of exercise. You sleep better. You eat better. And you feel better about yourself.

So why are we blind to our need to exercise?

Why We Don't Exercise

You may have a number of reasons for not exercising, and you may or may not be conscious of them. See if any of these ring a bell for you:

1. It won't help me. It won't actually make a real difference in my health. I think I am one of those humans who actually cannot benefit from exercise.

2. It will be uncomfortable. I won't like it. I hate being sweaty, hot and out of breath.

3. It's not that important. After all, I'm so busy. To this excuse I pose the popular question, *"What's better for your busy schedule? Exercising once a day, or being dead all week?"*

I'll cover the motivation topic again in the last chapter of the book, but here's a sneak preview:

You are never going to be motivated to exercise the way you need to exercise in order to be as physically fit as you need to be in order to live the quality life you want to live.

At least not at the beginning.

But you will become motivated – much more motivated, in fact, once you are well on the path toward being physically fit. That's because motivation feeds itself and when you don't offer it any food at the beginning (i.e., you don't exercise) that motivation doesn't have enough nourishment to live on its own.

So you'll have to radically accept this truth: it simply won't work to wait around until you feel like exercising. Feeling like exercising regularly is never going to happen out of the blue.

See, when you were young, your parents got you to do the stuff you were supposed to do. They provided the motivation for you to do things you did not want to do. Clean your room. Eat your broccoli. Save some money.

Now that you are a grownup you have to provide the rules for yourself, only you don't want to. So you don't. You have this idea that you get to choose anything you want and STILL have the same outcomes you used to have years ago. In your youth it felt so constraining to be told to do stuff that now you resist your own self when you tell yourself to do stuff, even when that stuff is going to increase your happiness.

It's like there's a three year-old somewhere inside you who's still demanding ice cream for dinner, and in the mistaken belief that you are being kind to yourself, you give in. After all, you hate feeling like you're forcing yourself to do anything.

That's because you have not yet learned how to kindly encourage yourself to do what's in your best interest. (It's definitely not too late! More on this in a later chapter!).

Eventually, when you're somewhere around 40 years old you run into a hard brick wall and realize that the outcomes you thought would magically happen have not actually happened. See, if you quit parenting yourself and let yourself indulge all day, the days and weeks turn into twenty years of self indulgence. And you end up with an addiction, or two or three. Perhaps you aren't addicted to cocaine (let's hope not). But you are almost assuredly addicted to something. Sugar? Coffee? Fighting with your partner? Watching TV?

Whatever it is, this addiction takes up your time and energy and keeps you from being fit.

Exercise helps. Exercise will heal your mind and your heart. Exercise will help you feel better about yourself, and it will help you be kinder to your loved ones. And exercise will help you get rid of that addiction, too. One study found that people who exercise (training by lifting weights) were twice as likely to stop smoking as compared to a control group that did not exercise but instead watched health videos for the same amount of time per week.[42]

As John Ratey, MD says in his book *Spark*, "...exercise is the single most powerful tool you have to optimize your brain."[43]

It's Not About How Much You Weigh!

I strongly encourage you to find reasons to exercise beyond wanting to lose weight. Losing weight is a good motivator for some people, but often once the weight is lost, the exercise is reduced, that is unless you fall in love with it and don't want to give up having all that fun! And the overall benefits of exercise go much, much further than mere weight loss.

By the way, for women in particular, short-term exercise alone (without dietary changes) is not going to bring on significant weight loss. Not understanding this, I remember one summer when I was very committed to weight loss through exercise. I went to the gym regularly and I worked out hard. I gained 14 pounds and didn't lose an inch. I did not make any dietary changes, and in fact I'm pretty sure I ate more because I was hungrier. I gave up when September came because I was so discouraged that I hadn't lost any weight. A few months later a fitness expert told me that if I'd just stuck with it, I'd probably have started to lose weight.

There's a study that looked at overweight women who exercised for 12 weeks and made no dietary changes. They didn't lose any significant weight. I did the same thing, and gave up. I wonder what would have happened in the study

> *Losing weight is a good motivator for some people, but often once the weight is lost, it's easy to reduce your exercise unless you fall in love with it and don't want to give up having all that fun.*

(or to me) if it had been a six month exercise program.

One final note before I detail some interesting things exercise will do for you: ladies, if you are exercising with a partner and that partner is a man, try your hardest to ignore how much more easily he will lose weight and gain muscle compared to you. It's not your imagination, and it is seriously annoying. Knowing to expect that difference between men and women regarding the immediate impact of exercise may keep you from giving up and drowning your frustration in a dozen red velvet cupcakes.

10 Things Exercise Will Do For You!

1. Exercise Creates New Brain Cells

Back "in the day" the conventional wisdom was that, once you lost brain cells, those dead cells, unlike other cells in the body, would never regenerate. Most people, even fairly recently, are still misinformed that brain cells are "one-time only" cells. The message was and often still is, "Brain cells don't grow back so, for heaven's sake, don't do anything to kill them!"

But now we know the brain does make new brain cells. It's a process called neurogenesis and we've only really known about it since 1997, far too recent for this information to have made it into most school curriculae. And it was only in 2007 that we were sure neurogenesis happened in humans.[44]

Not only does exercise spur the brain to create new cells, it also sets off the production of the ultimate new brain cell nourishment: Brain-derived neurotrophic factor (BDNF).

BDNF is a protein that is considered to be a nerve growth factor. It's found throughout the brain, but is primarily located in areas that are important to learning, memory and higher thinking[ee].

Interesting, isn't it, that exercise is such a boost for BDNF[ff] levels? We tend to separate exercise from intellectual pursuits, but here we see how intimately connected they are. Without exercise, you are at an intellectual disadvantage.

BDNF strengthens the connections between neurons, thereby building cell circuitry and nourishing cell functioning. One of the brain areas that is particularly rich in BDNF is called the hippocampus, and it's a critical area of the brain for functioning related to emotion and memory. Since the hippocampus is part of your brain's emotional circuitry, BDNF can be a link between physical movement and emotion.

2. Exercise Reduces Depression

An interesting study conducted at Duke University explored the connection between exercise and depression. Duke researchers found that 30 minutes of brisk exercise three days per week was just as good at lowering depression as medication.[45] Not only that, the study

---

[ee] It's also found in the retina and in your saliva, among other places.

[ff] But note that BDNF levels drop due to air pollution exposure, so when you are exercising amidst heavy traffic, you may not get quite the BDNF boost you are hoping for.

participants who simply exercised (as opposed to taking medication only, or exercising plus medication) had a much lower rate of relapse. Just 8% of exercisers had a return of depression, but in the groups that included medication (both medication only and medication plus exercise) the relapse rate was much higher: 38% and 31% respectively.

Exercise increases levels of BDNF, and BDNF boosts production of a neurotransmitter called serotonin. Serotonin is the neurotransmitter involved in thinking, feeling, sensitivity to pain, sleep and hunger. This neurotransmitter is strongly associated with depression and self-esteem, and is the neurotransmitter most frequently targeted by antidepressant medication. Furthermore, decreases in BDNF are associated with depression. Patients with mood disorders like depression and anxiety, or patients under a lot of stress have lower levels of BDNF in their blood. Patients with stress-induced depression show less BDNF in the hippocampus.[46]

Other studies have also found that exercise improves depression,[47] even if only a little bit. But some of the studies that showed exercise had a relatively small effect on depression also included people who might have exercised as little as half the time they were supposed to.[48] This is not a problem with the exercise intervention — it's a problem with adherence to the intervention. In other words, if you don't do the treatment, you can't say it didn't work.

Finally, depression is also associated with an atrophying hippocampus.[49] Since BDNF can increase new cells in the hippocampus, thus reversing this atrophy, it seems even more clear that exercise is a great way to treat depression. In fact, I consider exercise to be the most effective treatment for depression out there!

3. Exercise Also Relieves Anxiety

Anxiety is related to depression and most people with depression also experience anxiety (and vice versa). One study shows how exercise can help students with physical symptoms of anxiety – the kind that are often associated with panic attacks. Researchers split 54 students who did not normally exercise into two groups: one group worked out at a high intensity and the other group worked out at a low intensity. Both groups felt reduced levels of anxiety. The group with higher intensity exercise saw the reduction in anxiety faster, and even more interesting, they felt less afraid of their physical anxiety symptoms as early as after the second session of exercise![50]

Now, one of the difficulties people with panic attacks face is that any number of physical symptoms may become interpreted as signaling a potential panic attack, often setting off panic when it may not have occurred otherwise. So, if high intensity exercise can begin to reduce fear of panic attacks in a mere two sessions, I'd say that's great news!

What about those who don't necessarily struggle with panic attacks, but who struggle with the long-term anxiety which has traditionally been associated with personality type? Again, the research comes up very positively in favor of exercise's power to reduce the kind of anxiety that's "just a part of you" and not necessarily situational. Overall, exercise is one of your best bets for resolving mental health difficulties.

4. Exercise Helps You Learn

The brain changes as a result of what you tell it. In that sense you can change your brain just like you can change your waist size. What you put into that brain is what you get out of it.

In one study, volunteers who exercised for three months showed a 30% increase in newly formed capillaries (blood vessels that will nourish new neurons) in the hippocampus, one part of the brain that is strongly associated with memories and emotion[51].

Stress, on the other hand, limits your ability to be creative. Exercise is well known for decreasing general stress. Under high levels of chronic stress, your hippocampus begins to atrophy and levels of BDNF decrease. But the good news is that exercise can protect people from the loss of BDNF caused by stress in addition to nourishing the hippocampus.

Another study showed that people learn vocabulary words 20% faster following high intensity exercise than after low intensity exercise or after resting. Not only that, high intensity exercise also led to larger increases in BDNF and neurotransmitters[52] as compared to lower intensity exercise. I think that a 20% percent increase in learning is a big deal. It's a whole day of school out of a week. Your ability to remember and process new information increases significantly when you exercise. But do take note that you can't learn very well while you are in the very midst of exercising at high intensity. That's probably okay with you. I don't personally know anyone who memorizes vocabulary words while sprinting.

After that sprint, however – watch out! You are primed to learn.

5. Exercise Increases Creativity

Cognitive flexibility is the ability to switch gears between different kinds of thoughts, and the ability to think about multiple concepts at the same time. For example, a person who can go from analyzing why a toaster is not working to discussing the similarities between authors Kevin Hearne and Jim Butcher without a hitch would be a person of cognitive flexibility. The more cognitive flexibility you have, the better you are at learning.

Cognitive flexibility is also a huge component of creativity. Much of the creative act is that of integrating different pieces of knowledge in new and unique ways. This requires cognitive flexibility as a core practice. And exercise increases it.

Nearly 100 adults participated in a study of exercise and cognitive flexibility. Those who were randomized to the study group did either 3-4 days or 5-7 days per week of aerobic activity. The control group did 0-2 days. (Do you think the control group might have done more exercise than you do?! Time to take a look at what you are doing to your body!) After a 10 week period, researchers found that the more physical activity you do, the more cognitive flexibility you demonstrate.[53]

You don't even need 10 weeks of exercise to see improvement in your cognitive flexibility! Another study showed that participants' capacities to shift thinking, find new answers to questions, and engage in creativity (all hallmarks of cognitive flexibility) were improved after just one 35 minute treadmill session[54].

Here's yet another angle from which to think about this: studies of dancers show that moving to irregular rhythms improves their brain plasticity (the ability of the brain to form alternative and new connections). Perhaps when they are used to moving with regular rhythm their brains stop having to work as hard, and new connections are not as likely to be formed. But when the body starts moving to irregular, unexpected rhythms, the brain has to work to create new connections. This kind of work gives the brain practice in making new connections and thereby improves brain plasticity. The act of learning through movement is more powerful than asking the brain to do something creative without adding body movement. These dancers reaped heightened brain functioning as well as more finely tuned technique, all because the brain benefits from bodily movement.

6. Exercise Reduces Overall Cortisol

Cortisol is a hormone that your body produces which spikes in response to stress. Cortisol is essentially an anti-inflammatory hormone, and one of its effects (in addition to waking you up in the morning) is to reduce inflammation in the body. A little bit of cortisol is useful in dealing with occasional stress, but a lot of cortisol is a problem and affects your body adversely. For example, when you have chronically high levels of cortisol, you become more insulin resistant and your immune system doesn't work as well. Also, you crave more carbs and fats while simultaneously slowing your metabolism. Although while you are actively exercising, your short-term cortisol levels increase (because that's what cortisol does – it helps you get moving), regular and consistent exercise lowers your overall cortisol level.[55] Not only does exercise help manage cortisol better, but it also increases the production of other important neurotransmitters like serotonin, norepinephrine and dopamine.

It is key to do exercise that isn't damaging to your body – so we're not talking about running a marathon. What we're really after is reducing inflammation and stress. To get these good results, think about working at 70% of your maximum. That way you can maximize the positive effects of cortisol in the body. For example, did you know that cortisol increases glucose concentration in your blood so you can have easy access to energy right away? It also helps repair tissues that are broken down through exercise. So although cortisol levels can be indicative of stress and inflammation, do not oversimplify by concluding cortisol is always bad.

Similarly, don't avoid movement or stress out of a misguided sense that doing so will help reduce your cortisol levels. Even if you regularly work out for an hour a day, if you spend all your other work hours sitting at a desk, you are still at an elevated risk for inflammation-related problems, like Type II Diabetes and heart disease, despite your workout! Long periods of just sitting are never good for you.

Consuming caffeine is one method people use to get themselves moving, but you want to be careful with it. Caffeine raises your cortisol levels higher than normal throughout the day, and caffeine will result in higher than normal cortisol levels during exercise (especially for men). One way to counteract that potential problem is through increasing your omega-3 fatty acid intake. Omega-3 fatty acids have been shown to lower cortisol levels as well as reduce inflammation. Try to move toward ingesting less coffee, and more fish, flax seed, sea buckthorn or chia seed. Please understand, though, that I'm not saying increasing your omega-3 intake is a good enough counter to your caffeine intake. Your best health bet is to find a lifestyle that results in sufficient energy without caffeine. Embracing the three-legged stool approach can create that energy.

Your body has what's considered to be a "set point" for cortisol functioning, meaning that cortisol is released when a certain level of stimulation (anxiety, anger, etc.) is reached. Having a low threshold for anxiety (you get anxious quite easily) and a low threshold for cortisol release means that your body is releasing cortisol more frequently than if you had a higher set point. Regular aerobic activity can work to help calm you so that your body can handle more stress before cortisol is released. Thus regular exercise can help to change your cortisol set point. Seriously, how cool is that?!

7. Exercise Creates Better Sex

Oh yes. Not only does exercising make women feel better about their bodies and boost their self-esteem, but it also helps men perform the way they'd like to perform. Men in their 50's or older who exercise vigorously for about three hours per week are only about 1/3 as likely to experience erectile dysfunction as compared to men who exercise very little or not at all.[56]

8. Exercise Improves Attention

Attention and attention problems have a lot to do with the brain's executive functioning. Executive functioning is a term to describe brain operations that work like the way a corporate CEO decides what needs to be focused on in company operations at any given moment. Executive functioning is just like upper-level management, and not at all like filing alphabetically. So when a person with attention problems has trouble remembering the list of things his wife asked him to buy at the grocery store, but then has no trouble paying attention to the latest action movie, it may be that it's about executive functioning and not because he "just doesn't listen" to his wife! (Well, it may be independently true that such a guy doesn't listen much to his wife, but that's not the relevant issue here.) For true ADHD/ADD sufferers, this is a brain issue, not an issue of respect, organization or self-centeredness.

Dopamine is one of the neurotransmitters that is involved in directing the brain's attention to what the brain determines is important. The kinds of things individual brains find important vary from person to person. Dopamine calls your attention to the things that your brain specifically finds important in any given moment.

I have a child who qualified for an Attention Deficit Disorder (ADD) diagnosis, but for a long time I did not think that he had ADD when I saw how he was able to hyperfocus for long periods of time on particular things. Was the diagnosis wrong? Just because he could happily read an 800 page book didn't mean that his brain was able to process and attend to all the other input in his life with the same amount of motivation and attention. It wasn't because he was choosing to be difficult, and it wasn't because he didn't understand how to be organized or how to use his time strategically. He understood all of those things. The executive functioning part of attention happens way before the person can decide on any particular organization or strategy. The idea is, "If I don't see it, I can't fix it." Attention is derailed because the brain is signaling that something else is more important in that moment. So people with ADD tend to miss things. A lot. And attention tests show that people with ADD do have brains that function differently from people who don't have ADD: there is 10% less activity in the prefrontal cortex which is the part of the brain that is responsible for directing and regulating behavior (and using logic, identifying consequences, etc.).

The surprise was that as I observed my son's attention difficulties over time, I had insights into my own behavior and recognized that I actually had many of the same struggles. Realizing this helped explain a lot about both me and my son.

Both my son and I have found that excellent brain nutrition makes a big difference as we deal with our ADD — so big, in fact, that many of our ADD symptoms are negligible when we practice good habits of brain nutrition. Nutrition includes sleep and exercise as well as healthy eating habits. And since in this chapter we're talking about exercise, let me be more specific about what this means:

Exercise increases the levels of neurotransmitters dopamine and norepinephrine, lower levels of which are implicated in ADD. Most of the drugs that target ADD symptoms are drugs that increase these neurotransmitters. Exercise does the same thing. And regular, habitual exercise helps the brain far more than occasional exercise does. Consistent exercise makes us less likely to react irritably or out of proportion to problems, and helps us shift our attention more smoothly from one thing to another.[57] Interestingly, research has shown that boys appear to need more exercise for these kinds of improvements as compared to girls.

Exercise helps calm down the brain's amygdala, which is a part of the brain responsible for starting the fight-flight reaction as a result of strong emotion (think of lots of fear or anger). People who exercise are less likely to overreact to situations, which is another typical manifestation of ADD. Of course, emotional overreaction can also be a problem for people without ADD, so don't imagine that everyone who overreacts must have ADD! By the same token, however, exercise will definitely help everyone whose amygdala tends to overreact, no matter the root cause.

An important point here is that merely increasing norepinephrine and dopamine levels isn't always enough, nor is it always a good idea. Having more of these substances in the system is not always better, and there is a point at which too much of these neurotransmitters create negative effects. That's why the neurotransmitter increases from exercise are going to be more useful than those from medication. Your body will not create "too many" of these neurotransmitters through exercise, although it's surely possible to get too many of them through medication.

The best thing for you to do is just exercise and pay attention (!) to how much your exercise affects your ability to...pay attention.

9. Exercise and Heart Disease

We all know that aerobic exercise helps decrease heart disease, and here is part of why that is: As you breathe more deeply, exercise gets the blood pumping through the body at a faster rate. This increases production in the arteries (the arterial endothelium, to be exact) of a substance called nitric oxide. Nitric oxide is what helps relax blood vessels, inhibits the formation of blood clots and holds back the development of the plaques in arteries that are associated with blockages and consequent heart disease. Also, faster-flowing blood helps arteries resist the formation of new blockages. So exercise in order to produce more nitric oxide!

A recent comparison of drugs and exercise for heart disease found there was no difference between the effects of exercise or drugs in preventing heart failure, stroke, coronary heart disease and diabetes.[58] One of the conclusions drawn by the media[59] upon the publication of that study was that since drugs and exercise seemed to have equal impact, scientists should change the way they structure studies so exercise is always included as a comparison.

Take a second to think about the side effect profile of both choices: exercise vs. medications. I'll take exercise any day!

10. Exercise Improves Overall Motivation

If you are human, you've struggled with motivation. Sometimes it's really hard to get yourself moving, to stop procrastinating and to get started on your daily tasks. Exercise can help change all that. Regular exercise changes it even more thoroughly than occasional exercise, so be sure to make life changes that create dependable exercise in your life as a matter of habit.

Exercise also improves self-efficacy, your ability to believe you can do hard things. This is essentially motivation. People who are exercising feel more self-efficacy than people who do not exercise and that fact is another illustration that you must start doing a behavior before you feel like doing it. You might be one who could react to this information with a sense of frustration, discouragement or even outrage: "It's not fair that you have to do it before you feel like it!" Let me assure you that you will feel like exercising once you start doing it regularly. It will get easier. But in the beginning, there is no substitute for the hard work of starting. Part of your increase in self-efficacy once you exercise regularly is that you'll have just experienced multiple instances of getting yourself to do something hard, something you didn't want to do. This action increases self-efficacy.

When, as a result of regular exercise, you have changed your life so that your attention is better, your creativity is increased, your mood is good and you have generated a sense of self-efficacy and power, then you will find yourself more motivated than you ever thought you could be! You feel better about yourself. You will be much more likely to follow through on what you need to do to accomplish your other goals. These effects can start showing up the first day!

Find something you like, something you can see yourself doing regularly for years. Figure out a way to create the space in your life for exercise, and then treat the time it takes like a really important meeting. Don't let yourself let it go for anything.

Chapter Nine

Inflammation

T here are any number of popular movies and stories wherein the hero or heroine has to face danger and desperately wants a weapon for defense. What would James Bond do without his government toys? What would MacGyver do without duct tape? So too, our bodies need to defend themselves against the many troubles we are up against: bacteria, viruses, injuries, parasites, tumors, and all kinds of other villains.

Lucky for us, our bodies are amazing and we have highly specialized means to defend ourselves against each of these onslaughts. Of course, these defenses work much better when our bodies are healthy.

Inflammation is key to our defense.

Inflammation is how living body tissues respond to injuries. When under control, inflammation does an amazing job of promoting healing by creating conditions in which healing can occur efficiently. Inflammation is awesome.

In the short term.

However, inflammation that has become excessive, out of balance and out of control becomes a problem. Such inflammation becomes damaging and disease-promoting when it becomes chronic.

That is to say, when our bodies are under a constant onslaught of stress whether it's from bacteria, cell damage, excess hormones, or whatever, the body becomes chronically inflamed in its attempt to fix these problems.

If you think about the effects of eating fast food every day, and what that does to your gut and brain, you can see why a body can develop chronic inflammation. It's as if every morning you ask someone to punch you in the nose. Pretty soon you see a red, swollen nose all the time. It becomes your constant.

But the good news is that, just as you can stop asking someone to punch you in the nose every day, you can also work to stop chronic inflammation. You can change lifestyle patterns that contribute to this kind of inflammation.

I see a number of young adults in my practice who are just learning about how to take care of their bodies. Unfortunately, their youth gets in the way. Because their bodies are young and resilient, they can handle much more abuse than anyone who is much older. A 20 year-old can pound hamburgers and a shake, down a soda and some chips and then stay up until one a.m. without significant suffering the next morning. If I did that, I'd be a mess for two or three days. Young bodies don't tell as much truth about the damage done by poor eating and sleeping as older ones. As a result, young people often don't understand how important good nutrition and healthy sleeping are, because they don't suffer the consequences of poor sleep and poor nutrition with as much pain as those same unhealthy behaviors will cause them later in life. So youth understandably develop poor habits because, thanks to their inherent youthful resilience, they *can*. Then suddenly they turn 30 or 40 and their bodies slam into the brick wall of "See? See? You can't get away with this anymore. Welcome to the pain, my friend."

What Happens During Inflammation?

In acute inflammation — the kind nature designed to help your body — the body accomplishes two goals: it creates a barrier to protect against the spread of infection from the injury, and it heals damaged tissues. Pain, redness, swelling, and warmth occur, often resulting in some loss of function. Even though the injury site may look like something has gone terribly wrong, this inflammation process is designed to help your body.

Any injury will trigger an immediate and *acute* response, a short-term means of managing the situation. Let's look at this with an old-style[gg] military battle analogy.

[gg] Last century. Modern warfare is something I have no understanding of.

To begin, imagine the setup. First responders (white blood cells) constantly prowl through your bloodstream awaiting any attack from any direction. In addition to first responders, the bloodstream also carries fluid called *exudate* that can quickly be sent to any attacked location. Exudate is like the military supply water that carries everything necessary for a successful first response.

The enemy attacks. Boom! Chemical mediators tell the nearest blood vessels to increase their permeability so that within seconds, exudate fluid and white blood cells can leak out of the blood vessel and quickly arrive at the scene of the attack. In fact, capillary (very small blood vessels) pathways are quickly built to the attack scene so that repair materials can be delivered. It's kind of like the Army Corps of Engineers building roads to the attack scene, but in this case it's endothelial cells building capillaries and creating the pathways.[60]

The first responders to arrive at any attack or injury are generalists, and as such, they devour all potential invaders. They aren't looking for any particularly specific threat yet — they will take down anything that remotely looks like a threat. As these first responders are devouring enemy cells, exudate is also filling the injury site with salts and fluid to carry in repair supplies as well as to bring in

Exudate Fluid consists of:
High concentrations of salts
Immune system proteins (immunoglobulins)
Fibrin
Neutrophils
Lymphocytes
Macrophages

more specific fighters. Blood flow to the attacked area is increased, and the body tissue surrounding the injury consequently begins to swell, stopping the blood flow and thereby keeping the fighting contained. This swelling traps enemy attackers so they don't spread. Warmth (created by increased movement of the blood), redness and swelling are all results of the rush of fluid and blood cells to the injury site and their activities once they arrive.

The Immune System Manages Inflammation

Each defensive wave of fighters brought to the attack scene by the exudate is carefully orchestrated by a command-and-control structure housed in the immune system and staffed with excellent communicators, strategists, spies and analysts. They've received information from the first responders, describing what the attack looked like and what is required to fight a good fight. The immune command-and-control center sends out messenger cells called *cytokines* that are used to signal when to start inflammation and when to shut it down. Cytokines also help communicate how strongly to ramp up the attack (how much inflammation is needed).

Blood vessels leading away from the injury site are essentially sealed off, preventing the loss of cytokines and white blood cells and other healing molecules from the scene, as well as making escape more difficult for various microbes, etc. The area around the injury now has only one door open and the exit door shut. At this point the injury site is filled up with cells that can work to repair and rebuild tissue, as well as destroy infection.

This process can occur in minutes or hours and can last for days if necessary. It depends on how severe or lengthy the attack is.

While exudate is creating swelling to trap the attackers, the special force teams are getting into formation. *Complement* is a group of proteins carried in the exudate that act together to initiate inflammation. It's like a squad of Navy Seals. Specialized proteins link together in groups of nine. The ring-like link formed by complement is called a *membrane attack complex*, or *MAC*. I like to think of it as the MAC attack. MAC controls the movements in and out of the cell of substances like calcium ions which contribute to cell death.

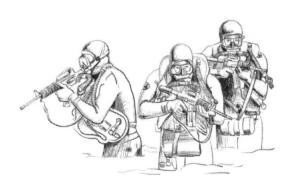

Other specialty fighters appear. *Lymphocytes* (among them T cells and B cells) arrive to more specifically target enemy cells. *Macrophages* and *monocytes* march in, devouring enemy cells and assisting the body in even more specific attacks against the invaders. The immune system analysts take notes about microbes involved in the attack, updating the immune system's memory files so if that particular kind of attack ever comes again in the future, a ready-made response can be more quickly deployed.

Eventually when the repair job is finished and infection is no longer an issue, the body signals for the exit door to open. Then all the exudate — that healing fluid bursting with pro-inflammatory cytokines and macrophages — is released. Now that it's no longer needed, the swelling goes away.

During healing, the body uses pain signals to help you act in ways that are protective to the injured tissue.

What we've seen so far in this military analogy are all the signs of acute inflammation (swelling, heat, redness and pain). Now you likely better understand the parts they play in healing. Of course, how well your body can achieve its ultimate goal of healing depends on how well your cells are able to regenerate[hh], and what kinds of injuries that were sustained.

I think it's fascinating how swelling, pain and warmth are so very useful in healing, and not just an annoying part of the injury trauma. Often

---

[hh] Needless to say, this is dependent on your overall health.

Some of the Players

Cytokines *are proteins that act as messenger chemicals.*
Some turn on inflammation and other cytokines turn it off.
Pro-inflammatory cytokines include IL-1, IL-6, TNF-alpha
and TNF-beta. The most common anti-inflammatory
cytokines are IL-4, IL-10 and IL-13. In research studies,
when herbs or other substances lower levels of TNF-alpha
and IL-6, you know that the herb can be considered anti-
inflammatory.

Excitotoxins *are another family of molecules that create*
cell death. Glutamate is a example. It's important in its
regulated sphere of influence, but too much glutamate
results in neuron death, through the action of letting
calcium ions into the cells through MAC.

Prostaglandins. *There are some prostaglandins that are*
pro-inflammatory (PG2) and some that are anti-
inflammatory (PG1 and PG3). PG1 and PG increase oxygen
flow and decrease pain.

Macrophages *are cells produced in the bone marrow that*
play a critical role in initiation, maintenance and resolution
of inflammation . This process, called phagocytosis, is one of
the functions of macrophages and helps clear infected, dead
or otherwise unwanted cells from the body.

Microglia *are the brain's macrophage cells, and while*
normally they are inactive, when activated they act like
macrophages do, and engulf or devour enemy cells. For
example, nerve cell injury due to glutamate (think MSG in
your Chinese food here) can induce long-term microglial
activation in the brain.

we mistake good health as equivalent to having no swelling, no heat and no pain in our bodies. So instead of addressing the causes of these signs of healing, we seek to get rid of the symptoms. We reduce swelling, heat and pain with anti-inflammatory medication; we lower fevers, we take pain relievers, etc. The natural bodily defenses, however, can be crippled by these misguided attempts. The body's best defense troops were using inflammation to solve an injury problem, and now they have been artificially denied this method. It's similar to the military's being grounded and not allowed to fight back. Without inflammation, the body is simply not as capable to efficiently kill microbes or heal from injury.

When we learn to better understand what the body is doing, we see that some of our conventional "stop the symptoms" responses to problems (for example trying to immediately reduce swelling or lower a fever) may not always be as helpful as we think.

Chronic Inflammation is the Real Problem

Many Americans are getting on board with the idea that inflammation is a root problem that underlies most (perhaps all) chronic disease. Certainly there is a wealth of research that now supports the role of inflammation in disease states such as heart disease, Type II Diabetes, Multiple Sclerosis, Alzheimer's disease, bowel diseases and even dental decay. However, the standard response in much medical practice is still to look for a Magic Bullet solution, a panacea in a pill. Statins, for instance, are an anti-inflammatory solution[61] that have been advertised to lower cholesterol, but evidence of their unintended negative effects continues to mount. Another example is the baby aspirin many Americans have been advised for decades to take once per day as a way of lowering the risk of heart disease. Our Magic Bullet is that we think we just need to take an anti-inflammatory pill to fix the problem rather than resolve the multiple causes of systemic, chronic inflammation.

It's not as though our body is just *imagining* that there's a problem and deciding to create chronic runaway inflammation for no good reason. There is indeed a problem.

It is the *chronic* inflammatory response that is problematic. When inflammation continues beyond its intended period of time, cell and tissue damage can result. Chronic inflammation can be a result of acute inflammation if the body can't stop the injury. We mentioned cytokines — the messenger cells that signal both when to start inflammation and when to shut it down. It's the imbalance in these two signals that can leave inflammation ongoing. Research has shown us how complex the interplay between acute and chronic inflammation is[62], but it might help to think of this complicated interplay as if it were disrupted communication on the battlefield between the attack site and the immune system's command and control center.

Pro-inflammatory cytokines are messenger cells in our immune system that help kill invader cells (using oxidative chemicals like hydrogen peroxide). They respond to signals to keep up the cell killing and the other pro-inflammatory activities. They also respond to signals that call for a "cease and desist." When these cytokines don't get a signal to stop, they can continue to kill cells in the body, and eventually the cells marked for death are not just invader cells. For example, cytokines might begin attacking cartilage in your knees, resulting in unchecked joint inflammation. You might try to resolve this situation with an anti-inflammatory medication, but you are only taking care of the symptom and not the root problem. There is an underlying reason the body is continuing to signal the presence of invader cells and continuing to release pro-inflammatory cytokines.

As another example, macrophages that are supposed to be deactivated by anti-inflammatory cytokines (messenger cells, specifically including interleukin 10 or IL-10 and transforming growth factor beta) are sometimes not deactivated and therefore continue to send out pro-inflammatory signals. Because the immune system is interdependent, one cell action can set off other cell actions. For example, when macrophages don't get the message to stop, and continue their work of killing enemy cells, they also stimulate the activity of more fighters called lymphocytes, small white blood cells that include B cells, T cells and natural killer cells.

So, poor communication between vital healing components in the cells resulting in non-deactivated macrophages or cytokines, can be one path to chronic inflammation. Other paths include injuries that cause ongoing damage resulting in constant repair processes, persistent infections, toxin exposure or problematic autoimmune responses.

One example of the kinds of problems that can occur due to chronic inflammation is the excessive production of collagen tissue. Collagen is kind of like spackle — it's a repair attempt of the body that can result in scar tissue when healing doesn't fully occur. Did you know that scar tissue doesn't always happen on the surface of the skin where it's visible? Invisible scar tissue can interfere with the normal functioning of the surrounding tissue. It then becomes, to continue our military analogy, a barrier to good cell communications.

Chronic inflammation is particularly damaging to blood vessels.[63] The endothelial layer of the blood vessel (the single thick cell lining inside the vessel) is what blood flows directly over, and is therefore very vulnerable to whatever is in the bloodstream. Some examples of substances that potentially damage the endothelial layers of blood vessels are: microbes, excessive blood sugar, low oxygen, high levels of acidity, and tobacco-related toxins. Obesity creates belly fat that produces its own inflammatory cytokines. Periodontal, or gum disease, also releases acids and infectious toxins from the mouth into the bloodstream. Even household cleaning supplies can trigger inflammatory responses. The resultant damage to blood vessels is a primary cause of heart disease.

Why You're Chronically Inflamed and What You Can Do About It

Let's talk more about that example of knee inflammation. When the acute stage of injury has passed or there is no apparent injury visible, figuring out why the body might be stuck in the inflammation loop can be very complicated, so often we just give up. We tend to think our knees either get injured or that age creeps up on us and we just wear them out. We imagine that chronic inflammation "strikes" apparently out of the blue. We feel relatively helpless about our ability to do much about the persistent and painful inflammation, so we're tempted to go get an injection, but evidence shows injections don't actually help much[64]. There is, however, a fair amount of evidence that our lifestyles have quite a bit to do with maintaining healthy joints. This next section will detail many lifestyle factors that contribute to chronic inflammation.

Our Pro-Inflammatory Lifestyle:

Diet Is A Big Factor!

Let's start with a crucial fact: sugars are pro-inflammatory. A long term study of nearly 50,000 men showed that fructose (e.g., in sweetened soft drinks or fruit juices) was associated with a significant increase in risk of gout, the most frequent form of inflammatory arthritis in men. Soft drinks and fruit juices were analyzed separately, and increased risk factors were found in both.[65]

Of course, general nutrition really makes a difference in joint inflammation. A cross-sectional study of older women found that those with rheumatoid arthritis were significantly more likely to have historically eaten a far less nutritious diet compared to women without rheumatoid arthritis[66].

One reason your physician may not tell you all about the benefits of a healthy diet is that she or he may not believe it's a realistic intervention for you. That's to say, your physician is betting you won't actually do the dietary work consistently, so there's little point to actually telling you about this potential solution. (Another reason may be that he or she is entirely unaware of these data). Yes, consistency is a hard thing to learn. But it's possible, so don't give up. Perhaps the way you've been doing it is what's not working. Stick with me throughout this entire book and we'll get through this together.

A healthy diet is in itself anti-inflammatory. You almost don't need to try hard to identify specific anti-inflammatory foods if you're eating mostly plants. General plant food is anti-inflammatory and is full of antioxidant activity. If you want one specific example, (and a few "high dollar words" to use with your friends), try this on: Galactolipids (which consist mainly of special kinds of fat with even bigger dollar names like monogalactosyldiacylglycerols and digalacto-syldiacylglycerols) are found in a wide variety of edible plants and are not only anti-inflammatory but also anti-tumor.[67]

Galactolipids are in beans, peas, kale, leeks, parsley, spinach, asparagus, broccoli, Brussels sprouts, chili peppers, bell peppers or pumpkins[ii].

[ii]Each of these foods contain a particular galactolipid named: 1,2-di-O-alpha-linolenoyl-3-O-beta-D-galactopyranosyl-sn-glycerol.
Seriously, did people use long names like this before "cut and paste?"

Exercise Reduces Inflammation

Exercising is another great anti-inflammatory activity. I know, I know, your knee hurts, so you want to be smart about this. But it's still true that exercising (for almost everyone) will make that knee feel better. But, please don't underestimate how important it is to exercise correctly. I could talk your ear off about how simply changing the alignment of my feet resulted in a drastic reduction in knee pain. I thought I was doing exercise the right way, and a new trainer showed me I was not[jj]. Now I can walk down stairs with no knee pain whatsoever, most of the time. (I don't hesitate to mention that I also included healthy eating and sleeping, as well as some great anti-inflammatory plants[kk] such as Chinese skullcap, boswellia, curcumin and noni fruit in the treatment of my own knee pain).

Quality Sleep Reduces Inflammation

Sleeping plays a huge role as well. Not getting enough sleep is pro-inflammatory, and stressful. Getting enough sleep acts as an anti-inflammatory. When you get enough sleep, your body has a chance to heal from the stress of the day, release human growth hormones and generally take care of the business that being

---

[jj] I constantly worked on aligning my feet so they were parallel to each other and not pointed out at all. This was hard to do while walking down stairs, but I took the extra time to do it. I also did a lot of barefoot walking, rolling my foot on a baseball and a superball, and I changed to minimal style tennis shoes. Thank you, Michael Page.

[kk] Thank you, SolleNaturals

---

awake gets in the way of. On the other hand, poor sleep raises your overall level of cortisol. Chronically high levels of cortisol are damaging to the body and can result in impaired thyroid functioning, lower levels of growth hormone, and increased abdominal fat.

Stress Increases Inflammation

Stress is pro-inflammatory. Stress alters how cortisol works. When you're stressed, you have more cortisol in your system (to help you respond to all the tigers your limbic system thinks are about to attack you). When there's chronically more cortisol in your system, your body tissues lose sensitivity to cortisol and then those tissues can't regulate inflammation like they are intended to do.[68]

Pain-Reducing Meds Hurt Your Gut

Many people rely on ibuprofen to help them manage knee pain. But as you are probably seeing by this stage in your reading of *The Fix*, everything is connected. Knee pain isn't in a separate universe from the rest of the body, even though doctors may act as if it were. ("Ma'am, you'll have to go see a knee specialist for that pain. You can find her office right next to the gastroenterologist that you'll be seeing after you've been on that pain medication for awhile.") In 1999, one of medicine's top journals – the New England Journal of Medicine –published an article stating that NSAIDS (non-steroidal anti-inflammatory drugs such as ibuprofen) cause about 16,500 deaths *per year*, just from gastrointestinal side effects. Side effects like liver problems, blood disorders, vision problems, etc. are not limited only to those people who take NSAIDS long-term. These unwelcome challenges are risks from the first dose onward. Not only that, we also know that taking NSAIDS can delay tissue healing. After all, they interfere with the body's well-designed methods for healing damage.

But perhaps more importantly, we also know that taking ibuprofen decimates the friendly flora in your gut. And friendly flora (probiotics) are critical to reducing body inflammation. And so now we come to Big Idea Number Four:

Big Idea #4: A healthy gut biome leads

to a balanced inflammatory response.

Gut health leads to a balanced inflammatory response

There are about 100 trillion or so bacteria inside you that are beneficial to your body. They keep you healthy. They help digest food, they detoxify poisons, they are part of your immune system and they even act as a protective barrier on your skin and inside your body, keeping out the dangerous pathogenic bacteria. These helpful bacteria are called probiotics. Your body contains some unhealthy bacteria also, and probiotics keep these numbers down so that your health is not compromised. If you have about 85% good bacteria vs. only 15% bad bacteria, you are probably in pretty good shape. But most Americans have fairly unhealthy gastrointestinal systems. If you measure love by behavioral results, it becomes clear that we hate our guts. The levels of friendly flora (the probiotics that live in our gastrointestinal system) in our guts should be much higher than they typically are, and this problem only gets worse as we age.

- Our ability to produce sufficient hydrochloric acid to digest food well worsens as we get older, with consequent ill effects on friendly flora.
- We eat poorly (too few vegetables, too much sugar and flour, and too few fermented foods). Overeating, not chewing our food well, and not relaxing while we eat are associated with poor digestion and consequently reduced friendly flora.
- We use high numbers of substances that kill these beneficial microbes (antibiotics, antibacterial soaps, chlorinated and fluoridated water, pharmaceuticals, etc.)

As a result we end up with a decidedly-damaging overgrowth of unfriendly bacteria, viruses and fungi in the small and large intestines. Our immune system has to sweep in to fight much harder to control these problems, because the friendly flora that should have been in the gut to do the job are not there.

Such an overactive response from the immune system can trigger food allergies, and imbalanced intestinal bacteria can further damage the gut. The next paragraph details even more escalating problems which can result from the interactive effects of imbalances in the gut flora.

Food allergies cause not only increased inflammation but also problems in the absorption of nutrients needed to sustain good health. Gut functioning continues to become more problematic as soon as the gut cannot regenerate itself as well as it could formerly, and the GI system becomes even more permeable (this is also called "leaky gut"). Not only does this raise systemic inflammation, but it also allows problematic bacteria that should have been killed in the stomach to escape into the bloodstream where the bacteria can latch onto cells in the joints and soft tissue. The battle escalates, and now the immune system, continuing to try to get rid of this enemy bacteria, attacks it in the joints, resulting in further inflammation and pain. Now the person has pain in the knees and when they take ibuprofen to manage the pain, more damage results, for not only does this pain-killer destroy friendly flora, but ibuprofen is in itself damaging to the mucosal lining in the gut.

In yet a further example of the inter-connectedness of bodily systems in the big chronic-inflammation picture, bacteria may exist in the mouth or gut and actually cause inflammation in the joints. Unfortunately, an inadequate probiotic population may not be strong enough to kill that bacteria.

The big link here is between gut health and inflammation. That's the major message of this chapter. The health of your gut microbiome (that is, your population of probiotics or friendly flora) is your first line of defense against almost every health challenge, including inflammation![69]

Interestingly, evidence shows that the gut microbiome profile is related to obesity and that people who are more obese show different patterns of friendly flora in their guts than those of thinner folks. Not only that, but when obese people lose weight, their gut flora change and look more like those of thinner persons.[70] Children who are overweight also appear to have different gut flora patterns compared to children at normal weights[71]. We also know that gut bacteria influence how much nutrition people can extract from the food they eat[72]. Perhaps even more thought-provoking a fact to consider is that we now know that gut microbes influence the body's insulin resistance, which further influences inflammation[73]! If you stick to that memorable saying: "If it's white, do not bite," your gut microbiome will benefit as some unfriendly strains of microflora can be significantly reduced when the intake of refined carbs is reduced.[74]

The problem is not *only* whether or not there is enough friendly flora in the gut — it's also about the variety of friendly flora in the gut. Each of us are host to several thousand different species of bacteria, and in this case, more is better. Recent research published in the journal *Nature*[75] showed that people with more genetic variety in their gut bacteria were healthier in general. People with less variety in their gut flora were more likely to be obese, more likely to gain weight over time, had higher cholesterol and more insulin resistance. The researchers were able to identify certain strains of bacteria that were associated with higher overall bacteria variety and other strains that were associated with less variability. The strains[ll] that indicated higher variability are also anti-inflammatory probiotics whereas — you guessed it — the strains found in people with less variability are strains known to be pro-inflammatory and pathogenic. A related study[76], also linking inflammation to gut bacteria, showed that people who ate less junk food had more variability in their gut biomes, but the researchers also found that people with low levels of friendly flora to begin with were not able to increase their bacteria variability just by eating more healthy foods. So the solution is threefold: 1) you need more friendly flora, and 2) you need more variety in friendly flora, and 3) you need to eat more healthful foods.

Are you improving your gut health through absorbing the marvelous array of beneficial phytochemicals found in plant foods? For instance, phenols in grapes can help prevent pathogens like salmonella from growing in the gut, and the resveratrol likewise found in grapes benefits friendly flora while helping rid the body of problematic microbes.

Part of what the gut does is protect us from any dangerous pathogens found in the food we eat. Friendly flora and stomach acid are the fighters here, and when we reduce stomach acid to unhealthy levels and/or when we take

---

[ll] Faecalibacterium, Bifidobacterium, and Lactobacillus are the probiotic strains reported. Each of these names are family names; there are lots of kinds of Bifidobacterium, for example.

---

antibiotics and thereby kill probiotics, then we have systematically gotten rid of most of our immune system.

Quorum Sensing is Cool!

Probiotics do something called "quorum sensing" by which they are able to sense how many of their particular strain exist in the gut biome. When there aren't enough of their particular strain of probiotics, those probiotics simply can't take the kinds of helpful, pro-health actions that we hope for. Helpful bacteria can take action only when there are enough of them do those actions. You have to reach critical mass before you get the benefits you are looking for. The take-home message here is this: Don't give up. Even if you don't see any benefits to your intake of probiotics, it doesn't mean what you're doing is worthless. Perhaps you haven't yet reached critical mass.

It's amazing how many times we make a health change for a few days or weeks and then discard that change because it seems to us (in our impatience!) that it's not working. Give it time!

It all comes back to lifestyle. You either lead a pro-inflammatory lifestyle or a balanced and anti-inflammatory lifestyle. What you eat, how you sleep, whether or not you exercise, how much perceived stress is in your life and the extent to which you use pharmaceuticals all make a significant difference in terms of your ability to enjoy a body that has a beneficial gut biome. The central theme of this chapter is that better gut health leads to less systemic inflammation. In contrast, poor gut health damages the body's immune system and leads to inflammation which results in a damaged, inflamed GI tract which produces frequent painful gas, diarrhea or constipation, heartburn or reflux. It's not many easy steps from occasional gut inflammation to truly problematic systemic, chronic inflammation.

Take the Path to a Therapeutic Level of Doing

When we think of the mind and body as two separate things, we also become too comfortable in casually separating our eating, sleeping and exercise habits from our ideas about general health. We know there is some kind of a mind-body link, but we don't understand how all-encompassing and pervasive it is. Take the example we have used in this chapter: inflammation in the knee. If we don't understand the big picture I have been painting in this book about mind-body health, we might think that awful knee pain is just a sign that the body has gone haywire. When we think we cannot trust our body's responses or we somehow don't work "right" anymore, it's easy to feel that what we do has little effect on our problems. And so we continue to eat, sleep and exercise poorly and we have little belief that improving these "three-legged stool" activities will make a difference.

> *What I'm talking about is having more commitment to a course of action so that what you do will influence your outcomes because you're doing it enough.*

A similar thing happens in mental health. People start to think that their emotions are haywire. They think they cannot trust how they feel, that their brain does not respond to their "sensible" attempts to control their feelings. So, believing that their emotions are out of control, they become even more discouraged and vulnerable to a slough of worsening emotional baggage.

Therapeutic Levels of Change

We may find that the health changes we are trying to make are not effective. In dismay, we then protect our feelings by refusing to look objectively at how consistently we are actually doing what we said we'd do (vs. what we'd like to believe we are doing). Or, we may harbor faulty health preconceptions and we are so defensive about them that we aren't open to finding out more accurate information that might make us more likely to accomplish our goals.

For example, we're told to eat a healthy diet, and so we do what we *think* is healthy and it doesn't really work. The most likely problem is that what we're doing is not at a therapeutic level. In other words, our "healthy diet" may just not be healthy enough. For example, you may think you have a healthy diet when it includes meat sources of protein at every meal, or even every day. But animal products are generally pro-inflammatory. They are hard on your body. It's not that you can never eat meat; it's just that you have to recognize that eating meat will raise the acidity level of your body and create inflammation. If you choose to eat meat every day, the result will be yet higher levels of inflammation.

We just talked about variety in probiotics. We may think we are doing good things for our bodies when we eat yogurt, which is advertised as full of probiotics, but what was shown so powerfully in the research above is that in order to have a real impact on our health, the variety and amount of probiotics we ingest are critical. Eating a yogurt won't give you enough probiotics, either in terms of variety or amount. It may help a little but it's simply not enough to make a difference.

Here's another example: You might try to add a few servings of fruits and vegetables to your diet in an attempt to become more healthy. But a few servings a day won't be transformative. You need to make a definitive change , such that eating "mostly plants" (thanks, Michael Pollan) doesn't mean you eat 51% plants and 49% animal products. The point here is that in order to create a lifestyle that is anti-inflammatory, you have to *really* change your sleep, lower your stress level, increase your exercise and especially add more vegetables and fruits to your diet. Include lots of those beneficial secondary metabolites that help reduce inflammation and help get rid of free radicals. You have to fight fire with, well...plants.

Doesn't sound catchy, but it's the truth.

Here's a further example to underscore my point that, to become healthy, we need to make therapeutically effective lifestyle changes: Vitamin D and omega-3 fatty acids are two more examples of under-utilized anti-inflammatories. Vitamin D levels are inversely related to proinflammatory cytokines[77]. What this means is that Vitamin D can help downregulate your body's pro-inflammatory messages. People understand that Vitamin D and omega-3 fatty acids are generally supposed to be helpful, but they don't often experience supplementing with them as being transformative to their health. The primary reason for this is that they don't take enough in terms of quality and quantity. They aren't doing the treatment at a therapeutic level.

One of my favorite ideas from the herbal medicine approach is that you have to be more aggressive in your treatment than the disease state is in its attack. To continue this chapter's battle analogy, you're better off using "shock and awe" on your side rather than waiting for "peace talks" to work. If you're ill, you can't sit back and drink a cup of ginger tea, hoping that that alone will do the trick.

Take Responsibility for Doing Enough

Perhaps one of the most important points of this entire book is to encourage you, the reader, to take responsibility for your health, and to do it without getting sidelined by shame and guilt. What I'm talking about is helping you intensify your commitment to a course of action that will actually improve your health. Only when what you *do is therapeutically enough* can you have a chance at realizing your desired outcomes!

And this is Big Idea #5:

Big Idea #5:
Only when what you do is
therapeutically enough can you have a
chance at realizing your desired
outcomes!

Chapter Ten

Cardiovascular Health

H eart disease is not a cholesterol problem. It's primarily an inflammation problem[78]. This idea is hard for the average person to accept, particularly when he or she is someone who has spent significant resources, in terms of time, energy, money, effort and hope, to take cholesterol-lowering medications. There are a few psychological processes that underlie the difficulties people face in accepting the fact that heart disease is not a cholesterol problem:

Availability Cascade is a term for what happens when we hear something over and over and then believe it to be true because everybody's saying the same thing. It's a bit like propaganda, except that propaganda is usually thought of with more suspicion because propaganda is an organized effort to persuade people. The availability cascade just happens in a way that's more similar to the rise of folk myths.

Another psychological idea is that of *Cognitive Dissonance*. When a person does something that runs counter to his beliefs, it's hard for his ego to admit to being wrong and so he justifies his behavior instead and becomes "resistant" to seeing the truth of what really happened.

Finally, the *Backfire Effect* occurs when people are faced with new information. Instead of accepting it they more strongly cling to their old information. It's hard to let go of our ideas about how the world works. Letting go feels unsafe!

The science supporting the inflammation basis of heart disease clearly exists. You can see, however, why it takes time for people to become "ready" to hear what the science says. I am reminded of a quote a cousin of mine posted online:

"Practicing honesty, open-mindedness, and willingness keeps us teachable, grateful and humble. The difference between humility and humiliation can be the level of acceptance we have about the information we get."[mm]

We get a lot of information that is hard to accept. Life feels so much more free and vibrant when we are able to handle new information without instantly skewing it to match our current behavior. When you decide to reach out to claim

---

[mm] Pg. 6 *Living Clean* by Narcotics Anon.

all truth, wherever it might be found, your ability to remain humble instead of persisting in being a *truth gatekeeper* radically opens you to many growth possibilities.

It's time to become a butterfly.

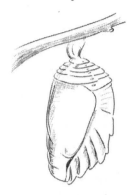

This idea is another riff on Chapter 3: that empiricism is really for open minds. Our cocoons may be safe, but they are also confining. Finding the truth is for open minds. It takes great courage to let go of our assumptions and instead let the truth speak for itself. Nonetheless, we must also recognize that we continue to hear everything nestled in the blanket of our previous experience. As we are more able to see and grasp the information in front of us with truly open minds, our subsequent experiences change us so we can more easily leave our blankets behind.

Veins, Arteries and Blood Cells

Cardiovascular health includes not only heart health, but also the health of our veins and arteries, and most particularly the thin layer of cells that line all of the above, called the endothelium. Our arteries and veins are made of smooth muscle and elastic connective tissue. Blood vessels are made to stretch. Endothelial cells have enough of a regulatory impact on the blood to be considered an organ. We often talk of the skin as being the largest organ, but it's actually the endothelium that is the largest organ in the body. The endothelium produces a high number of active molecules that regulate nutrients, hormones, and the permeability of blood vessel membranes. The endothelium also regulates which cells are permitted transport in or out of blood vessels, the blood cells themselves, and even blood flow.[79] These endothelial linings are constantly repairing and renewing themselves, as well as creating new blood vessels. So when the endothelial lining becomes inflamed, there is a pervasive negative impact on the body.

The take home message is this: You definitely want to protect your endothelial lining.

Damage to the endothelial lining can create high blood pressure, inflammation, blood that clumps together too much, and the buildup of plaque. These things continue to endanger the endothelium further, creating more damage. For example, the longer a person has diabetes, smokes or has high blood pressure, the more problematical endothelial functioning they have. And the more endothelial dysfunction, the greater the risk of a heart attack.

Essentially, it's a lot more complicated than the simple formula most of us casually think we understand: the higher the cholesterol, the greater the risk of a heart attack. No, it's not that simple at all.

Healthy Blood Cells

Blood, on average, is 55% fluid (90% of which is water) and 45% cells. This mixture carries oxygen, hormones and nutrients like glucose throughout the body. Hormones send messages to and initiate necessary changes in tissues throughout the body. Glucose provides fuel throughout the body.

Healthy red blood cells each have a negative electrical charge. Think about them as two magnets, both negatively charged. A negative and positive magnet will connect quickly, but two negatively charged magnets (or blood cells) repel each other and do not get stuck together. This is important for blood cells because some blood vessels – capillaries – are pretty narrow, and require the blood cells to enter one by one and not in big clumps. You see, when blood cells lose their negative charge, they tend to clump up. Too much clumping and it becomes hard for blood to move freely through veins and arteries, and consequently harder for the blood to carry needed nutrients and oxygen.

> **What are trans fats?**
> When hydrogen is added to vegetable oils, they become more solid, making them more appealing to the food industry. Foods then become less greasy and have longer shelf lives. Trans fats are also found naturally in meat and dairy products but these trans fats are structured differently and affect the body differently than industrial trans fats.

Healthy Blood Cells Require Healthful Fats

Another characteristic of healthy blood cells is their flexibility. Cell walls need

Your Total Cholesterol Count

Low density lipoprotein (LDL): *Cholesterol plus a protein. The very small and dense LDL type is problematic when it oxidizes because it can squeeze through the artery lining. LDL transports cholesterol into the arteries.*

High density lipoprotein (HDL): *Cholesterol plus a protein. This larger type of lipoprotein travels from body tissues like the arteries and takes cholesterol back to the liver to be recycled so it can go to other tissues that need it.*

Triglycerides: *The main factor in fats and oils; a blood lipid.*

Lipoprotein(a) or Lp(a): *This is LDL type cholesterol plus a protein called apoprotein a. Elevated levels of Lp(a) are a very strong risk factor for heart disease.*

to be elastic and flexible in order for the blood cells to squeeze through tight capillaries without breaking. Flexible cell walls have a healthy layer of fat (phospholipids) to aid their bending. Here, then, is one of the first things you can do to improve your overall cardiovascular health: eat the right kinds of fat. Ideally, your cells are able to build walls out of essential fatty acids but if those fats are not available, they'll take what is available. And if that means they use the fats from the burger you ate last weekend, so be it.

Since the fat that provides that layer around the cell is what determines how flexible or fluid the cell is, you'll want to make sure your cells are built out of high quality essential fatty acids. Cells membranes that contain fats from trans fats sources will not be as flexible as cell membranes made out of essential fatty acids; they will be limited in their ability to let necessary materials move easily in and out of the cell. Unhealthy membranes mean the cells can't hold nutrients, can't hold their electrical charges, and won't respond well to messages from the rest of the body. So do whatever you can to make those cell membranes healthy. Be sure you're eating plenty of essential fatty acids (omega-3's) and plenty of antioxidants (vegetables and fruits).

Low Fat Diets Aren't Necessarily Healthy

Many people believe that eating a low-fat diet is one of the most important things they should do to improve cardiovascular health. But experts disagree. A Harvard Heart Letter (November 2011) regards a low-fat diet as last in place as far as its positive impact on cardiovascular health. The letter also reported that people who follow a Mediterranean diet are likely to have lower LDL cholesterol, lose weight and lower their blood sugar, blood pressure and inflammation markers like CRP (C-reactive protein). You can now see that your blood cells desperately need plenty of essential fatty acids, so clearly what you need is not a low-fat diet in general, but rather a diet that's low in damaging trans fats and high in health-promoting fats like omega fats. A healthful fat diet simply does not include industry-created trans fats[nn].

[nn] Shortening and margarine are prime examples of trans fats.

Lowering Cholesterol Doesn't Guarantee Better Heart Health!

Perhaps one of the most misunderstood health topics these days is cholesterol. Cholesterol has become quite the villain and has been unfairly maligned as the biggest risk factor or cause of heart attacks. We all "know" that cholesterol levels of 200 mg/dL or higher are considered "bad" and put us at risk for heart disease. The Mayo clinic website, for example, characterizes cholesterol levels of below 200 to be "desirable" and levels of the LDL (the "bad" kind of cholesterol) to be ideal or near ideal when they are between 100 and 139 mg/dL.

Yet a UCLA study published in 2009 refutes this kind of thinking pretty powerfully. Over half of all patients (59% of nearly 137,000 people) who were admitted to a hospital for a heart attack did not have high cholesterol, but instead had normal to low levels. Specifically, the average LDL level in all of these patients was 104.9 ± 39.8.[80]

So lowering LDL levels of cholesterol is not a guaranteed strategy for avoiding a heart attack. Add to this the fact that your risk of premature death from non-cardiac causes actually increases progressively as your cholesterol levels decrease.

In 2005 we knew that people over the age 65 with the lowest cholesterol levels were twice as likely to die each year as compared to people over 65 with the highest cholesterol levels.[81] Most of us know that women tend to outlive men. Women also tend to have higher cholesterol levels than men. In fact, when men and women have similar cholesterol levels, the women are no longer more likely to outlive the men.[82]

Almost all of the cholesterol your body contains has actually been made *by* your body. Very little of it comes from the food you eat. Your liver alone produces about 75% of your bodily cholesterol. Your brain makes some as well. Whether and how much cholesterol your liver makes is actually influenced by your glucose metabolism, not by how many eggs you ate for breakfast. Incidentally, this is why it makes no sense to think of diabetes as being a condition entirely different from heart disease. Once again, everything's connected.

Scientists Have Known This For Years

In 1990 we had information from the Framingham study and the Multiple Risk Factor Intervention Trial that clearly indicated that the effect of cholesterol on heart disease diminishes with age and is not related to heart disease in men who are over age 65.[83] People over 70 with higher cholesterol levels were *less* likely to die of heart attacks than people over 70 with low cholesterol.

Also in 1990 scientists reported a 10-year study of cholesterol levels and colon cancer which showed that the people who ended up getting colon cancer had cholesterol levels that were significantly lower than non-colon cancer patients. The people with colon cancer also had cholesterol levels that continued to decline, compared to the non-colon cancer group whose cholesterol levels actually went up about 2%.[84]

And this is not isolated information. A 1997 study of over 11,000 patients showed that those with low cholesterol had over twice the risk of dying of any non-cardiac cause[oo] than patients with higher cholesterol levels (over 160 mg/dL). Fine, you might say, but what about heart attacks? The risk of cardiac death ended up being the same in both groups![85] Having low cholesterol simply wasn't a protection against a heart attack, and was actually a risk factor for any other cause of death.

So here's a crazy idea you may not have considered before: Cholesterol must do something useful for you after all!

> *The Mediterranean diet includes eating lots of fruits, vegetables, grains, beans, seeds and nuts as well as healthful portions of olive oil. Very little red meat is included, in addition to small portions of fish, poultry and dairy. It's not about eating tons of olive oil; it's about eating tons of vegetables and fruits*

Benefits of Cholesterol

Cholesterol is part of what makes up cell membranes. Cells need cholesterol for their own protection and to help them function optimally. Cholesterol is also needed by the brain and for the production of hormones like estrogen, testosterone and cortisol. Lower cholesterol levels are actually associated with increased risk of neurological problems such as dementia and

---

[oo] The most frequent cause of non-cardiac death was cancer.

Alzheimer's disease because cholesterol is what makes up the myelin sheath that insulates nerves and helps the nervous system communicate.

Cholesterol helps the body process and break down (emulsify) fats in the gall bladder. When you eat fats, your gall bladder releases bile to help aid you in digesting those fats. Cholesterol helps make up bile salts and therefore is used to help the body absorb all those good fats like omegas, vitamin E, olive oil, COQ10, etc. People whose gall bladders are functioning poorly, or who have had their gall bladders removed, have much more trouble digesting fats.

Cholesterol: Why Do I Want This Stuff?

Makes up cell membranes

Helps protect nerves

Forms part of myelin sheath

It's what vitamin D is made from

Helps your body absorb good fat (processing fat-soluble vitamins)

Building block for steroid hormones

Helps preserve brain function

In fact, your brain produces cholesterol, as does your liver

Cholesterol, Vitamin D and Serotonin

One of my favorite things to explain to people is that vitamin D is made from your own body's cholesterol. True story! The sun uses your body's cholesterol to create vitamin D. Kind of makes you feel good when you stand in the sun, arms wide to the sky, embracing the transformation of cholesterol into something you know you want: vitamin D.

Oh, and here's another good thing cholesterol does for us. Serotonin, that neurotransmitter we all associate so strongly with mood, is what we call cholesterol-dependent. You see, serotonin receptors (the things that receive the serotonin) require cholesterol to function well. When blood cholesterol is lowered, so is cellular cholesterol and consequently the number of serotonin receptors is decreased. More cholesterol equals more serotonin receptors. This fact helps explain why it is that when cholesterol is lowered, the risk of suicide and violent death increases.

Cholesterol is critical to healing and repairing cell damage. Remember, cholesterol helps keep the cell walls flexible, thus helping with overall cell functioning. It's very important. That's why your liver is so good at making it. When you have damaged cells, you need cholesterol to repair those cells, thus the liver gets the signal to make some cholesterol. Then the liver releases that cholesterol into the bloodstream so cholesterol can get to the damaged areas and begin to help make new, healthy cells.

Plaque

There are specific bunches of plaque that are worse than others; the size or age of the plaques do not seem to matter. Some plaques harbor a core of dead cells that set off dangerous clotting when the plaque bursts and the dead cells are released. These kinds of plaque are found to be dependent on a particular protein and are identifiable by the way blood flow indicates stress (detectable by MRI).

You may also believe that the more plaque and artherosclerosis (the fatty plaque deposits on your artery walls) you have, the greater your risk for a heart attack. But it's the rupturing, not the number of vulnerable plaques that is the problem.

Arteries can become blocked without rupturing, and at the same time, plaque rupture does not always cause blockage of the artery. So although these two events are linked (thrombosis and rupture), one can happen without the other, and you may not know either has happened depending on how complete the blockage is. Sometimes rupture happens and the detritus from the blockage is simply reincorporated into the plaque.

What does seem clear is this: when you have damaged arteries and oxidized cholesterol, you are creating the conditions for a heart attack or stroke.

damages the delicate oils, quickly turning them rancid (or oxidizing them). That's why you use olive oil on your salad, and not in your skillet.

If you want to cook in oil, use a stable oil that tolerates heat well without becoming oxidized. Raw, unrefined cold-pressed coconut oil is ideal.

In general, healthy cholesterol is not a problem in your body — it's a necessary building material for healthy cells travelling through your bloodstream. So it seems that one reason some people may have a lot more cholesterol than average flowing through their bodies is that some people's bodies need a lot more repair than the average. Your body may be suffering from inflammation in many places, so your liver is producing and releasing more cholesterol for cell rebuilding. It's the underlying inflammation and long-term damage to the endothelium that are the real problems. And cholesterol that is damaged, or oxidized is an associated problem. We'll consider that next.

There's another reason you might have more cholesterol flowing through your blood than what might be optimal if you were as healthy as you could be. You may not have enough friendly flora in your gut biome. These probiotics are part of your body's cholesterol management system.[86] They eat cholesterol, for one! Probiotics break down cholesterol molecules and use them for food. Probiotics also generate acids that reduce liver production of cholesterol. Finally, probiotics play a role in stimulating the liver to make more bile acids, which help in cholesterol metabolism.

Heart Disease is about Inflammation

So what actually causes heart disease if it isn't cholesterol? You already know the answer if you've been paying attention: inflammation. And in order to understand inflammation and heart disease, we really need to chat about plaque.

What is Plaque

Plaque isn't the same thing as cholesterol, although most of us talk about it as if it were. When most people talk about cholesterol building up in their arteries, they are really referring to plaque. Plaque is thickened areas in the blood vessel walls. The thickened areas are primarily made up of cholesterol, collagen, calcium, and fat. But here's the kicker — the most problematic cholesterol that is found in plaque is cholesterol that has been damaged by oxidation. It's this damaged, oxidized cholesterol that is the deeper problem in the blood vessels, because oxidized cholesterol requires healing — and inflammation happens as part of the body's attempt to heal.[8788]

As you remember from the last chapter, inflammation promotes healing by creating swelling and signaling white blood cells to come help. Various factors combine to make blood thicker so it can clot, and to help blood vessels constrict, so you don't keep bleeding. Collagen (a structural protein like glue) is produced so that, eventually when you heal, you may have a protective scar formed over the formerly damaged area. When arteries are damaged, the same process occurs within the artery. In this case, however, that same scar is known by a different name: plaque.

There are times when damaged cholesterol gets into a damaged artery wall and creates more inflammation. That's not hard to imagine, given that oxidized cholesterol travels throughout the body. Bear in mind, the more oxidized cholesterol you have, the greater chance this is happening. The body thinks the oxidized cholesterol is something harmful (thanks to the inflammation) and so macrophages come to the rescue and surround the cholesterol, drowning it in an attempt to destroy it. When macrophages and cholesterol become bound together like this, these swollen masses are called foam cells[pp]. The foam cells hook up with calcium and some other substances in the blood, and become plaque, the plaque that clogs your blood vessels. Remember, the body was trying to heal itself, but it was doing the healing with what was available and that was damaged (oxidized) cholesterol.

So it's not cholesterol that causes heart attacks. Cholesterol is trying to repair damaged arteries. Magic Bullet thinking assumes that since higher cholesterol levels are associated with heart disease, it means that cholesterol causes the problem, and that therefore the way to solve that problem is to decrease cholesterol levels. Now you can understand why the real problem is the underlying inflammation that damages the cardiovascular system. And you can also see how useless it is to simply lower your cholesterol level. It's as though you were telling your liver to quit making materials for healthy cells!

Fire Department Analogy

Here's an analogy. There have been a lot of houses catching fire in your neighborhood lately. So there are lots of firemen and fire trucks and sirens in the neighborhood. Very busy! And all the people whose homes have burned are moving

---

[pp] My personal theory is that the scientist responsible for naming this had just eaten marshmallows.

away. The city officials take a look at what's going on and they get alarmed[qq]. It's a huge problem that so many people are moving away. So they decide that the cause of the problem is all the noisy firemen and fire trucks. They get rid of the fire department.

Hmm.

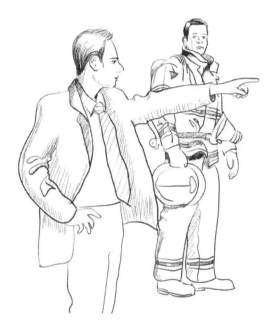

To extend the fireman analogy, think of it this way: sometimes the fire department mistakenly employs firemen who are secretly pyromaniacs. So those firemen (think oxidized cholesterol) really *are* a problem, and when you get rid of the fire department, it may be that the overall number of fires is reduced, thanks to getting rid of those few that were pyromaniacs. So

---

[qq] I know, I'm hilarious. Alarmed. Ha ha.

it wasn't the fire department, or even most of the firemen that was the problem. It was those few damaged firemen.

Lowering cholesterol doesn't affect the amount of arterial plaque in your body. It just lowers your cholesterol, and we've seen that just lowering cholesterol doesn't fix the problem. If you want to reduce plaque, you have to reduce your levels of inflammation and oxidation.

Magic Bullets for Heart Disease

Next time you meet with your doctor about your cholesterol levels look again at Magic Bullet thinking. In this case, Magic Bullet thinking is a real problem, not only because it inspires people to frantically lower their cholesterol but it also makes people spend a ton of money on products that are likely to damage their bodies and increase their risk of death.

Magic Bullet thinking is a great way to function when being chased by a tiger (run or die! run now!) but not so great when we are trying to figure out how to solve a complex problem. Heart disease is a complex problem, and you can't solve it by merely lowering cholesterol, just like you can't solve osteoporosis by increasing calcium or drinking more milk, and you can't fix diabetes with more insulin. But when you say "death by heart attack!" people get a little nervous and start making judgments with emotional "all or nothing" thinking. Hence the deceptive Magic Bullet solution for "death by heart attack": just lower your cholesterol.

What Can I Do To Help Myself?

As an alternative to magic bullet thinking, I suggest you fully engage yourself in pursuit of the three-legged stool approach to total body health: eat right, sleep right and exercise. If you smoke, stop. If you live or work with smokers, find a way to eliminate your exposure to smoke. If you drink, be sure it is only in moderation, and if you don't drink, don't start. If you have diabetes, take care of it.

Sleep is a big deal. Research has shown that people who get sufficient sleep have a lower risk of cardiovascular disease events (stroke, non-fatal heart attack and fatal heart attack), even beyond the lower risk that a healthy lifestyle will get them.

Eating food with lots of antioxidants is very important for heart health as these chemicals help neutralize damaging free radicals and reduce oxidation throughout the body. In addition to fruits and vegetables, many medicinal herbs are high in antioxidants. For example, yerba mate tea was shown to increase plasma and blood antioxidant protection in patients with high levels of cholesterol and triglycerides.[89] Vitamin D has been shown to help with pretty much every function in our bodies, and that's true for its efficacy in reducing heart disease, too. There were some initial cautionary arguments that vitamin D increases calcification, but this was based on an animal study where the animals were give 2.1 million units of vitamin D. Since that amount was a lethal dose, of course it created problems. So don't take a million units of vitamin D! A much lower, but still therapeutic dose may help reverse hardening of the arteries.

Magnesium also has a tremendous impact on body health. It helps reduce calcification of the arteries, lowers cholesterol (remember, more cholesterol is an indication of more inflammation; magnesium is a potent anti-inflammatory) lowers triglycerides, raises HDL cholesterol and inhibits

---

Supplements that help Cardiovascular disease:

Consult your physician first

Vitamin D: *You'll want D3 and it's important to take it with K2. Don't take too little. Get a blood level drawn (25-hydroxy). Many people can take 5,000 units per day without a problem.*

Magnesium: *This mineral is crucial, particularly in balancing calcium and helping calcium play its role. Bioavailable sources are what you want.*

Vitamin K *reduced heart disease mortality by more than 50% in people who consumed high amounts from foods (think spinach and broccoli).*

Vitamin C *keeps cells in good repair. Low levels of vitamin C can more than double calcium buildup in coronary walls.*

Hawthorne *has been shown in a Cochrane review to significantly help heart functioning by reducing oxygen needed by the heart, improving exercise tolerance and reducing fatigue and shortness of breath.*

Note: This information is not intended to treat disease, but is for educational purposes only. Please see your doctor for the treatment of disease.

---

the formation of artery-blocking kinds of blood clots.[90,91]

Finally, if you are especially working to reduce the risk of heart disease in your life, be sure to read the parts of this book that deal with anxiety, stress and self-compassion. Stress creates inflammation in and of itself. Learning how to live life in such a way that you are not experiencing stress is crucial. Remember that stress is your perception of what's happening, not necessarily how busy you are or how many problems you have.

Avoiding heart disease comes down to the basics, like it does with every health problem we run into. Eat right, sleep enough and exercise well. Live with love[rr], laugh well and forgive, and your heart will always be with you.

[rr] If you thought of the phrase, "Live, Laugh, Love," I'll have to take away your man card. Sorry.

Chapter Eleven

Type II Diabetes

Most people think of Type II diabetes or what people call *insulin resistance diabetes* in fairly simplistic terms. They figure that a person with Type II diabetes got the disease because he or she ate too many donuts and watched television instead of doing something more active. And in fact, this is a truly excellent road to getting Type II Diabetes. However, it's not the only road, nor does it guarantee diabetes, and this is why understanding Type II diabetes requires an understanding of the whole self rather than a separation of mind and body.

Sounds familiar by now, doesn't it?

Perhaps you anticipated this next sentence: thinking simplistically about Type II diabetes (that the problem is too much sugar and the solution is to adjust insulin levels) is really just another classic case of Magic Bullet thinking!

The overall purpose of this chapter isn't to have an in-depth discussion about how diabetes works, but rather to highlight how mind states are connected to what we tend to think of as body diseases. The causes of diabetes are much more complicated than overeating and inactivity. There are significant and far-reaching mind-body interactions that also contribute. We'll take a look at how stress, depression, anger and hostility are involved.

As you can probably guess by now, cortisol is implicated in all of these "mind" states (you know I say "mind" with quotation marks because it's not separate from the body), showing us one clear link between emotions, psychology and diabetes.

Your conventional doctor is probably going to tell you that Type II Diabetes is a disease that prevents your body from properly regulating your blood sugar. You might learn that you don't make enough insulin any more to manage the amount of sugar in your blood. Therefore you either need to control your blood sugar with diet or medication, or you'll have to go on supplementary insulin for the rest of your life.

As truths go, this one is so reductionistic that it creates a lot of inaccurate assumptions in treatment. People start thinking that they can eat that chocolate cake. After all, they are on insulin so it won't matter. Not so.

To believe that you can keep eating the standard American sugar diet as long as you stick to your diabetes medication is pure fantasy.

(Actually to believe that you can eat the standard American sugar diet and stay remotely healthy at all is likewise a fantasy!)

Of all the diseases that we look at in this book, Type II Diabetes may be the most simple and the most complicated at the same time. It's a very treatable and preventable problem and in this sense it is simple because it is so fixable. However Type II Diabetes is also much more than a blood sugar problem. Dysregulated blood sugar arises from many sources and creates many other problems. Type II Diabetes is complex. The "fix," however, doesn't have to be.

First we'll talk about the relationship between Type II Diabetes and various emotional states, and then we'll talk about some ideas for the "fix".

Type II Diabetes is Depressing

Nothing like getting hit while you're already down, is there? It's easy to imagine that having Type II Diabetes would be depressing, and indeed having Type II Diabetes does increase the risk of becoming clinically depressed[92], but not just because having diabetes is a big downer. Once people with Type II Diabetes become clinically depressed they are also at an increased risk of complications like circulation problems, foot ulcers and even limb amputation[93]. Treating that depression, however, leads to better outcomes for Type II Diabetes.

Risk goes both ways, however. Having depression significantly increases your risk for Type II Diabetes (studies say from 40% to 60%[94,95]). Basically this means if you are or have been clinically depressed (that is, either you were diagnosed with depression by a doctor or your answers to a depression questionnaire would have shown that you were clinically depressed) you are more likely to develop Type II Diabetes.

The severity of your depression and anxiety also plays a role. The more anxious or depressed you are, the higher your risk of developing Type II Diabetes.[96]. You don't even have to have had an actual episode of depression or anxiety – you just can have what's called a depressive temperament. A depressive temperament is a personality that is gloomy, self-critical, and pessimistic. This kind of thinking, feeling, perceiving and living results in having more trouble regulating blood sugar[97].

You can see the mind-body connection here.

Emotions, Cortisol and Type II Diabetes

When we have emotions such as fear (anxiety, stress), anger, or intense sadness, we release a chemical called cortisol[ss]. Cortisol is intended to help us — it creates the fight or flight reaction that helps defend us from danger. When cortisol is released it sends more blood to the muscles, increases the heart rate, and helps us be more aware of our surroundings (hypervigilance). Clinical depression is associated with increased cortisol and adrenalin release[98], even with chronically high levels of cortisol. Cortisol also raises blood glucose levels *and* makes our cells more resistant to insulin, thus

---

[ss] Incidentally, you know what also causes a release of cortisol? Eating sweets and too much meat.

keeping more sugar available for use in the blood. This is quite helpful if you have to fight a tiger. However, the system that releases cortisol doesn't really discriminate between tigers and modern-day stressors that aren't actually life threatening. So instead of fighting or running, we cope in other ways:

"Dude, hand me the cookies. I'm so stressed. Give me sugar."

Although most of us have experienced the carbohydrate cravings that result from stress, coping by eating sugar is one of the worst things we can do for our bodies while stressed. Researchers have found when people are stressed after a meal they have trouble regulating blood sugars. Interestingly, when people are stressed while fasting from food, their blood sugar shows much less dysregulation[99].

Stress, depression or anger – all of them can make us want to eat. That sugar coma or leaden feeling of absolute satiety is one of the most used (or abused) methods of numbing emotions known to man, perhaps second only to alcohol. And now you might be thinking, okay, I see there's a connection between stress eating and Type II Diabetes. But there's more of a connection here than eating cookies under the influence of cortisol. Even if you control your

> **What's Metabolic Syndrome?**
> *Obesity, high blood pressure and insulin resistance are all risk factors for heart disease and Type II Diabetes. When these risk factors occur together, it's called metabolic syndrome. Some estimate that over a quarter of Americans have metabolic syndrome.*

eating and don't reach for the candy when stressed, the emotion states of depression, anger, hostility and stress will still make you more vulnerable to Type II Diabetes.

Type II Diabetes and Anger or Hostility

People who are often angry or hostile are more likely to be insulin resistant or to have Type II Diabetes. There are a host of studies that show this relationship. Here's one I found particularly interesting: Researchers measured the hostility level of over 900 women living in Finland. Nine years later, the researchers took another look at these women. They found that women with higher levels of hostility 9 years earlier had a higher risk of metabolic syndrome and a higher rate of systemic inflammation. Even more interestingly, the behaviors that you'd think would significantly add to the risk of these problems, such as smoking, drinking, and lack of exercise, were outweighed by that nine-year higher hostility level. Sure, people who were more hostile did tend to smoke and drink, and exercised less, but whether or not they smoked, drank or didn't exercise, their hostility level ranked as the most important factor in predicting inflammation and trouble with blood sugar regulation[100].

The take-home message here is *not* that smoking, drinking and lack of exercise don't really affect your health. They absolutely do. However, hostility also affects your health in very profound ways. Learning to manage anger appropriately (that means managing anger without violence, alcohol, etc.) will bring tremendous benefits to your physical health. To reiterate, hostility increases your risk for metabolic syndrome which can lead to Type II Diabetes. Hostility is associated with chronically high cortisol levels, and it's been proven that too much cortisol and adrenalin lead to obesity and insulin resistance. There's no doubt that both obesity and insulin resistance are on the expressway that leads straight to Type II Diabetes.[101]

Type II Diabetes and the Workplace

Perhaps you think that stress is part of everyone's workplace environment and that workplace stress doesn't really "count" toward Type II Diabetes? Think again. Excessive overtime at work yields a 4-fold increase in risk for Type II Diabetes in Japanese men.[102] And may I just point out that Japanese men are a group of people with a decent reputation for relatively healthy eating?

In addition to excessive overtime, being burned out at work also increased men's risk for Type II Diabetes[103]. Tense working conditions are related to Type II Diabetes onset in women.[104] One interesting note is that general stress at work seems more predictive of Type II Diabetes in women than men. For men, but not for women, simple workplace stress (not burnout, not overtime) did not increase risk for Type II Diabetes.

Type II Diabetes and General Stress

Okay...so you aren't really an angry person, and you don't see your workplace as very stressful. But you're not out of the woods yet. General stress— the non-workplace kind — also creates elevated blood glucose levels even in people without diabetes.[105]

Type II Diabetes and Poor Sleep

There is also an interaction between sleep and Type II Diabetes. I'm not just talking about how eating cookies at 2 am contributes to blood sugar instability. Sleep is incredibly important and lack of sleep has serious implications for diabetes. Poor sleep quality impairs glucose metabolism, and makes you more hungry. This increases your risk for both obesity and Type II Diabetes.

Poor sleep leads to a rise in cortisol, which can result in chronic inflammation. Poor sleep has been linked to a pre-diabetic state wherein your blood sugar is higher than normal without being high enough to qualify for Type II diabetes. Often when you sleep poorly, you also experience carb cravings and you want to eat lots of simple carbs like bread and sugar the following day. Those cravings are an attempt by your body to get more energy to make up for the lack of sleep. But when a person arrives at a pre-diabetic state it's not simply because he or she noshed on sugar too much.

A study of healthy young adults found that after only three nights of poor sleep (the researchers selectively suppressed slow-wave sleep), these young adults became less sensitive to insulin, meaning that they needed more insulin to manage the same amount of glucose. Reduced tolerance of glucose resulted, and this metabolic state is one of the prime risk factors for developing Type II diabetes. These participants' poorer sensitivity was actually at levels similar to what would have happened if they had gained 25 extra pounds!

Processed Foods: Just Say No

Finally just one more thing, and I know this is kind of like kicking you while you're down, so brace yourself:

Bleached flour is a serious problem.

Chlorine gas is often used to bleach flour. Yum! When chlorine gas hits flour, a lovely byproduct called alloxan is created. Alloxan is a chemical that actually destroys beta cells in the pancreas. Beta cells are the cells that produce insulin. Alloxan kills them. Alloxan is actually so good at killing these cells that its use is a standard method for creating diabetes in rats for studies. The diabetic rats thus prepared for studies are even called "alloxan rats."[106]

Keep in mind that many products that wouldn't seem to need bleached flour still contain it. Grocery store brownies are a great example. They are known for being lusciously dark brown, but they contain bleached flour. This is because bakers often prefer bleached flour to unbleached flour because it's lighter in weight, making it easier to bake with, and it's more consistent in color.

This is Discouraging

Some of you might want to throw in the towel at this point. After all, it seems that everything you love is bad for you. Staying up late, noshing on ice cream while watching television, sleeping in instead of getting up to go to the gym, telling your boss off when you feel like it...all the things that we seem to think either bring pleasure or are simply normal human coping mechanisms are being condemned as giving a person Type II Diabetes[107]. But let's look at this concept of "pleasure" again, because there are multiple ways to experience pleasure in our lives. Could it be possible that getting to bed early, eating mostly plants, exercising daily and not holding grudges or getting angry are lifestyle choices that could actually become much more pleasurable than you might currently imagine?

Of course, in order to find out whether what I am suggesting here could be really true, you have to make those lifestyle changes and do those behaviors! Here's the crucial sequence: First, do the behavior, then you'll have the proof! This is the empirical method after all: we test the principles that make sense to us, we gather the evidence, and then we make what truly become informed decisions about whether or not to continue doing the behaviors we've been testing.

Okay, I Have to Change My Life. Now What?

We return to the three-legged stool approach (healthy eating, exercise and sleep) as a foundational basis for helping with Type II Diabetes (that stool fixes most of our problems, doesn't it?) as with everything else. In working with Type II Diabetes, these three legs are crucial, and if one or more of the legs are left out, the proverbial stool will not support our lives and health.

But, as we have seen in the studies cited earlier, there is another component to successful treatment for Type II Diabetes and this component is the mind. What we have learned about causative factors for Type II Diabetes is a tremendous example of "one thing leading to another." So our focus here turns to helping you figure out how to change your lifestyle in ways that will really work to reverse or prevent Type II Diabetes.

Sticking to a Plan

What we know about patient adherence (or compliance) with health practices to manage of Type II Diabetes is that it's pretty poor. Fewer than 20% of people with Type II Diabetes actually follow through on doctor recommended exercise. Many people want to believe they can just pop a few pills and continue with their old lifestyles. They deceive themselves into thinking they can "have their cake and eat it too."

Sadly, Type II Diabetes is a killer. And we know that if, as a Type II Diabetes patient, you're depressed, your track record for adherence to medical advice is going to be even worse. Adherence to conventional treatment is so time-consuming and difficult that it's incredibly dis-couraging. It never seems to end. In the words of a dear relative of mine, "I'd rather have cancer."

Many people with Type II Diabetes are deeply discouraged. They fear that what they might be doing to cope with the disease isn't really helping, they don't like the side effects of prescribed medications, they feel deprived, and they don't even have time to prepare better food choices, etc. Discouragement is a tremendous problem! But learning how to manage and alleviate discouragement is primary in a whole-body approach to helping diabetes. High levels of blood sugar don't just affect your body; they also affect your thinking and your emotions. And in yet another example of the circularity of causes and effects, all the evidence points to the fact that your thinking and emotions affect your blood sugar as well!

What Can I Do?

The message of hope is this: Type II Diabetes can be overcome. Start now. You can beat this. Here are some steps to take:

1. Take a good quality probiotic. Probiotics are not only associated with better emotional regulation, but also with better control of blood sugar[108]. Take the probiotic in the morning on an empty stomach and wait about 20 minutes before you eat breakfast.[tt] Include fermented foods in your diet, and stay away from substances that destroy your friendly flora (e.g., antibacterial soap, alcohol and sugar are three such substances).

2. Get some vitamin D3. If you're not taking vitamin D after reading the first few chapters of this book, start now. Vitamin D is associated with a lower risk of Type II Diabetes[109] and might be the least expensive and easiest thing to do. A

[tt]Stomach acid that is released when you eat food will result in a higher death rate for ingested probiotics.

good quality vitamin D supplement is one of your must-haves. Use D3, not D2 and get the kind with Vitamin K2. Even better than taking a supplement is to go make your own vitamin D by being in the sunlight.

3. Exercise. This is the number one thing you can do to help. Type II Diabetes responds incredibly well to regular exercise. If you skip this step, you are skipping perhaps the most important thing you could do to help your condition and you are far less likely to get better.

Wave Exposure for Food

1. Think about how hungry you are in general at the moment. Rate it on a scale of 1 to 10.

2. Now think about a food you love but you know is not good for you. Notice how you become more hungry. Rate your urge for that food on a scale of 1 to 10.

3. Distract yourself from the image of that tempting food. Do something else, think something else, etc. Set a reminder to come back to this exercise in about 30 minutes. (If it's close to meal time, you'll want to eat something but make sure it's not the food you have an urge for, rather, something good for you instead).

4. Now that you're back, rate your overall hunger again.

5. Imagine the wanted food item again. Rate your urge. Distract.

6. Repeat over and over and you will notice that your urge for that food will decrease.

---

4. Change your eating style. This is a long-term change and not a short-term diet. Here are a few ideas:

• Chew your food until you could practically drink it. Focus on taste. More saliva results in more easily digested food, better nutrient intake, less hunger and therefore less overeating. Less overeating creates better control of blood glucose.

• Eat slowly. It takes 20 minutes for the brain to start sending out signals that you can stop eating.

• Eat only until you are not hungry, and not until you are full. Awareness really helps with this part. It's easier to do this when you are eating healthy foods rather than sugary, fatty foods that override your good sense.

Variation on Wave Exposure:

Food in Front of You

1. You can try the same kind of thing with food right in front of you.

2. Place a desired treat in front of you and simply look at it. Don't eat it. Just notice how your urge for that food goes up.

3. At some point, that urge will plateau. Pay attention to your urge for the food so you can notice when you reach that plateau.

4. After the urge plateaus you will notice it drop. You can create another urge by thinking about how good the food would taste. If you do that, simply notice it again and wait for the plateau.

Try the wave exposure exercises (shown in sidebars) to manage eating that comes from urges not related to hunger. Instead of telling yourself that you simply just *must* become more aware of your eating and never eat to regulate your emotions, do some wave exposure. Repeat until you are good at it.

Alternatives to Conventional Treatment for Type II Diabetes

It is incredible how many plant substances are known to help lower blood sugar. It is easy to find evidence for them in medical literature. The insert on pg. 199 lists some of the plants that I found in a not very exhaustive search. Some are better known for their glucose lowering abilities than others. There are a number of products on the market that contain one or more of these herbs. Often these combinations can have a synergistic effect, providing more together than they would apart.

Remember, anything you do to specifically work on lowering blood sugar will work far better

---

A Non-Exhaustive List of Herbs With Blood Sugar Lowering Potential

bitter melon (also known as bitter gourd or Momordica charantia), berberine, cayenne, cedar berries (juniperis monosperma), cinnamon, comfrey, coriander, dandelion, fenugreek, garlic, goldenseal, gymnema sylvestre, licorice root, mullein, nopal cactus, panax ginseng, pterocarpus marsupium, salacia, uva ursi

---

when done in the context of the three-legged stool approach.   Just like adding insulin doesn't address the root cause of Type II Diabetes, adding helpful herbs also doesn't address that root cause.

But the most important thing you can do is to simply get started doing something. As you do one or two things well, these simple actions will increase your level of motivation and your energy to do even more.

It's not too late.

Chapter Twelve

Depression

Treating depression would be ever so much easier if I had a magic wand, but lacking that unrealistic alternative, it would be scads easier if depression didn't suck all the motivation out of a person. Not only does depression create feelings of sadness and despair, but it adds apathy and hopelessness to the mix. Depressed people have incessantly recurring thoughts and feelings such as "I don't care," and "Nothing will ever get better." Often, and understandably, such a person may even start to have wishful thoughts of death – the ultimate "get-out-of-jail" card — or so some are tempted to think. These thoughts just come with depression, and having such thoughts doesn't mean depressed people are crazy. Rather, these thoughts mean that experiencing depression (and

I mean real "clinical depression") is simply miserable. The depression feels unending. Most of the "suicidal ideation" that comes along with depression boils down more to a desire to escape and quit feeling so horribly bad than an actual desire to die. Since depression brings hopelessness and guilt, and messes up your thinking bigtime, depression will trick you into believing that the only way to quit feeling so miserable is to die. And herein lies much of the trouble, because depression is in large part a problem of *amotivation*, that is, a serious lack of motivation. If depressed people knew what to do *and* were able to jump up and do it, they could and would overcome depression much more easily. But a lot of the time depression makes the mind disbelieve that any possible way of addressing the sadness and despair will actually work.

Much of the information in this chapter focuses on how to improve brain health. Instead of giving depressed people a list of things to do in order to change (not a very effective approach), we focus instead on building brain health that will not only decrease depression, but also work to improve motivation. Trying to feel better by mere willpower is just about guaranteed to fail. Pushing yourself to "snap out of it" may yield a short term boost in motivation, but in the long run you often feel even more discouraged and unmotivated.

Part of my incorrigible optimism on this crucial subject is my belief that depression can truly go away—- and not come back. Most patients with "intractable" or "treatment-resistant" depression (depression that doesn't seem to go away, ever), or recurrent depression have had treatment that's been limited to psychiatric medication and/or "therapy." It's often unclear just what is meant when a patient says he or she has "had therapy" because the experience of having had "therapy" varies greatly. Even standardized therapies can look pretty different when applied by different therapists. I've found that about half of the patients I see have been on a mixture of psychiatric medications (usually the standard antidepressants, often augmented with anti-psychotics and anxiolytics) and many of them would strongly prefer to not take medication. The other half are not taking medication, and strongly prefer to continue to not take medication. Happily, there is an impressive amount of science-based evidence for effective mind-body depression interventions.

For a long time we have known that depression is intimately involved with what's commonly called the HPA axis, the connection between two parts of the brain, the hypothalamus and pituitary, and the adrenal glands. The hypothalamus manages how much cortisol a person normally has in the body[uu] and, in cases of threat, sends messages to the pituitary to increase stress hormones like cortisol. The pituitary then sends messages to the adrenal glands to release cortisol. Here's what we've learned: Depression causes the HPA axis to become more sensitive and overactive[110], so it more easily releases cortisol. Chronic stress also

---

[uu] Set point is the amount of cortisol that will create homeostasis for the individual; this amount varies depending on the person. Some people release more or less cortisol. Intake of food, exercise, sleep and past experiences all play a role in set point.

---

has this cortisol-increasing effect on the HPA axis Furthermore, traumatic experiences in life (especially at younger ages) can also affect the HPA axis, and even change the size of the hypothalamus.

The take-home message here is that depression increases the amount of cortisol circulating in the body. One of the things conventional antidepressant medications do, in addition to making the neurotransmitter serotonin more available, is to help regulate the HPA axis, and to lower blood cortisol. However, there are other very effective ways to treat depression without conventional antidepressant medication.

Depression and the Gut

So let's start with perhaps one of the more startling mind-body interventions for depression: probiotics. Each of us has about a trillion bacteria that live in and on our body, doing all kinds of good for us. These friendly flora protect us from non-friendly bacteria, they influence our immune system and neutralize toxins. (In this regard, you probably want to avoid using antibiotic soaps because although such products are killing bacteria, they are mostly killing your own defensive army.) Most of our bacteria exist in the gut where they help digest food, take care of toxic byproducts of digestion, regulate cell growth in the gut, and even produce vitamins B and K. We generally don't think of bacteria as related to mood, but what recent research shows is that ingesting probiotics can actually decrease anxiety and depression[111]. The bacteria in your gut transmit mood and behavior-regulating signals to the brain by way of the vagus nerve (a very long nerve that connects the stomach to the brainstem) and thus appear to have direct effects on brain chemistry. Perhaps even more surprisingly, this link between intestinal microflora and behavior-regulating signals is not new information; it was proposed over 70 years ago after research conducted on the connections between mood, gut bacteria and skin conditions.[112]

The implication here is that since what you eat affects the health of your gut, what you eat also affects your vulnerability to depression and anxiety. Instead of thinking of the food you eat as entirely independent of your mood, start experimenting by adding gut-friendly foods to your diet and eliminating some of the foods that create imbalance in your gut bacteria. Add plenty of raw foods, with a focus on green leafy vegetables, and foods with vivid colors. Avoid processed foods and sugar, and, in particular, avoid soda. If you have any trouble with leaky gut or irritable bowel, take steps to work toward healing these conditions. Antidepressants do have some anti-inflammatory effects, but it's much more effective to target the inflammation directly by changing your diet, adding probiotics and avoiding foods known to create inflammation and poor gut health.

Depression and the Mind-Body Connection

To my mind, depression is the illness that best demonstrates the powerful link between the mind and body. Depression in many ways is a "crossover illness," in that it has traditionally been understood as a problem in the brain or at least in the mind, but it includes a number of what appear to be strictly physical symptoms. I have seen a number of patients whose first indication of depression has been physiological. They may have felt fatigued, uninterested in eating, and unable to sleep (or unable to get up and feel awake) for some time before becoming aware that their mood is low or blue.

Here's what's really interesting: Although talk therapy can be very helpful and sometimes crucial for treatment of depression, some of the best treatments for depression are physiological. I like to use the below topics when I talk about depression with my patients. We talk about how each of these different areas specifically applies to that person's life. We are always careful to acknowledge that there is almost certainly something we are inadvertently leaving out, either because we have forgotten it or because we don't know about it. Here's the list:

Depression and Brain Health

I like to start with brain health. Helping patients understand that building a healthier brain is a large part of beating depression is not only evidence-based treatment, but it's also motivating. So many people believe that they can "should" themselves out of depression, or that there's something wrong with them because their willpower no longer works. Once you see that poor brain health is part of the problem, you have something more concrete to work on, and more importantly you realize that depression is not a personality failure. We begin by talking about two primary things here: vitamin D and omega-3 fatty acids.

People with low levels of vitamin D (levels that are less than 20 ng/mL) have more difficulty with their thinking, and are about 11 times more likely to be depressed as compared to people with normal levels of vitamin D[113]. I ask my patients to see their doctor in order to get a current vitamin D level (ask for the 25-hydroxy level) and then, if that level is low, to work with their doctor on raising their vitamin D level.[vv] Most physicians have been told that the minimum level of vitamin D that's considered normal is 30 ng/mL.[114] However, other experts recommend higher vitamin D levels (60-80) in order to access health benefits beyond basic maintenance of the skeletal structure.[115] Keep in mind, however, that levels higher than 100 ng/mL are dangerously high, although it's awfully difficult to get your levels that high.

When you talk to your physician, be sure to be well informed about vitamin D, in case your physician is not. One of my patients recently told me that her initial level of vitamin D was 16 ng/mL. She took some supplemental vitamin D and her next blood test showed an increase to 26 ng/mL. Her doctor told her that this represented really great progress and she could therefore quit taking the supplement!

Sunshine is usually the most efficient (and cheapest!) way to raise your vitamin D level, but

---

[vv] Consult with your physician before beginning any vitamin D supplements.

there are a number of reasons that sunlight alone might not work (for example, you may live at a latitude where the sun is not intense enough, or you may not be able to spend enough time in sunshine). If you decide to use supplements, it's important to take the D3 form of vitamin D, and to take the vitamin with dietary fat, since vitamin D is fat-soluble. If you take your vitamin D pill with orange juice and celery, you are pretty much wasting your time as far as the vitamin D goes (but that celery is great for stomach discomfort!) Adding vitamin K2 to your vitamin D regimen is very important, because it acts in synergy with vitamin D to help the D actually get to where it needs to go and not get stuck promoting artery clogging calcium. Guess what one of your sources for vitamin K is? Friendly gut flora. Green leafy vegetables are also good sources of vitamin K2.

I also educate my depressed clients about the importance of supplementary essential fatty acids. There is solid evidence that people with higher levels of omega-3 fatty acids (often referred to as PUFAs in the scientific literature) are less likely to be depressed[116], and that vice versa, people with low levels of these essential fatty acids are more likely to be depressed.[117] More severely depressed individuals have even lower blood levels of omega-3 fatty acids[118,119]. In fact, low levels of omega-3's are associated with negative moods even in people who don't qualify for a diagnosis of depression[120]. Low levels of omega-3's change the levels of both serotonin and dopamine, two of the neurotransmitters that play a large role in mood.

Phosphatidylserine (PS) is a specialized kind of fat that helps cells communicate. It also helps reduce depression, so you want to have enough of it. When you are deficient in omega-3 fatty acids, your brain has lower levels of phosphatidylserine.

Other positive impacts of omega-3 fats include help with concentration and less anxiety. In a study that compared medical students given omega-3 fatty acids versus a placebo, the students who received omega-3 fatty acids showed a 20% reduction in anxiety as well as a decrease in their IL-6 production (IL-6 is associated with higher levels of inflammation)[121]. It's important to note that these students received a large dose of omega-3 fatty acids (specifically, 2085 mg EPA and 348 mg DHA), actually far more than most people take when they add the average fish oil capsule to their regimen.

What these data illustrate is a review of the therapeutic dose idea we've covered earlier. When taking care of your body, you must reach a *therapeutic* dose of whatever supplement or activity you are engaged in. Taking a little bit of vitamin D may be nice, but it may not be nearly enough to help you in a way that you notice. Exercising a little bit is certainly better for depression than not exercising at all, but it may not be enough to have a significant effect on the depression. Similarly, you must take in enough omega-3 fatty acids in order to make an impact on depression and other health states.

Improving your ratio of omega-6 to omega-3 fatty acids is another tool for improving brain health. A healthy ratio is to eat only about four times as many omega-6 fats as omega-3 fats. Most Americans eat between 20 to 40 times as many omega-6 fats as omega-3 fats. A diet high in omega-6 fatty acids not only raises the risk of inflammation, but also raises the risk of depression[122].

Conversely, not only does an improved ratio of omega-3's to omega-6's reduce inflammation, but achieving that ratio in the body is associated with reducing depression. Interestingly, when you combine a lifestyle that includes too many omega-6 fatty acids with depression, both these factors (the omega-6's and the depression) have a *synergistic* effect. This means that when combined, they increase inflammation more together than they would individually on their own. For example, if depression yielded, say, a +2 on an inflammation scale, and too many omega-6 fatty acids yielded, say, a +3 on that same inflammation scale, then both of these factors taken together would yield something significantly higher than the expected sum of 5.

My recommendation here is to include omega-3 fatty acids in the diet, and reduce omega-6 intake by cutting back on meats and processed foods or anything that contains corn or soybean oil (soybean oil contains about 50% omega-6 fatty acids). Try switching to olive oil for salads (olive oil is only about 10% omega-6's) and coconut oil for cooking (about 4% omega-6's).

Fish oil has traditionally been the prime source for two of the omega-3 fatty acids that the literature has most frequently tied to good emotional health: eicosapentaenoic acid (EPA) and docosahexanoic acid (DHA)[123]. Many people have used flax seed as a plant substitute for fish oil, hoping that they can take in enough ALA (alpha-linoleic acid) to help their body make sufficient quantities of DHA and EPA from the

ALA. Sometimes this can be a little tricky, as the body is not very efficient at converting ALA to EPA and DHA. However, there is controversy in this area as well, and I think we don't have enough information about how ALA and other omega fats work in the body and the brain.

If you're looking for a plant source of omega-3 fatty acids, try sea buckthorn which already contains ready-made EPA and DHA as well as a number of other important omegas. Chia seeds also contain significant quantities of omega-3's.

Depression and Emotion Regulation

In my work with depressed patients we next talk about emotion regulation. Emotion regulation is your ability to manage and deal with your emotions, including your anger, your upsets, disappointment, sadness, grief and frustration. Part of what I teach in therapy is how to *tolerate* your emotions, and what to do to manage them. When I say tolerate, I don't mean "put up with." Rather, what I mean is to be able to fully experience your emotions instead of running away from them or getting rid of them. Most of us don't know how to have emotions because we learned instead how to get rid of them or how to avoid them, not because we are constitutionally unable to feel. Instead of experiencing our emotions, we try to get rid of them. Eating, drinking, drugs, buying shoes, sleeping, fighting, watching TV, and, well, being depressed: these are all ways to avoid experiencing emotions. Learning how to manage emotions can really help people be less vulnerable to depression. The key point here is that therapy can help you learn how to feel emotions without wanting to run away from them. Learning to experience emotions is a skill that can be one of the primary keys to success in life.

Depression and Cognitive Regulation

The related concept is learning how to manage your thinking. You may be stuck in thinking patterns that are full of what we call "cognitive distortions." For example, you might engage in "all or nothing" thinking where you inaccurately think in terms of "always" or "never." Such distorted thinking increases your vulnerability to difficult emotions.

If you have trouble with emotion regulation or thinking style, seek help. There are a number of resources. For example, competent therapists trained in Dialectical Behavior Therapy specialize in helping people learn to regulate their emotions. Psychologists who do CBT (Cognitive-Behavior Therapy) can help you with pervasive patterns of distorted thinking, and/or you can take a careful look at books like the classic *Feeling Good* by Dr. David Burns.

Depression and the Patient's Current Life Situation

Along the road toward holistically treating patients with depression, we next look at the patient's current life situation: his or her recent life events and other circumstances. When the current situation is taken into account, a person's emotions are almost always easily understandable. Sometimes patients are in the midst of overwhelming circumstances, or they feel stuck in situations that they don't know how to get through. Don't underestimate the impact of current situational stress on your physical and psychological functioning. Taking the time to strengthen the body while you learn to psychologically manage your current stressors is very important. Some of this management involves problem solving and learning what your emotions are telling you, and some of this involves sticking like glue to the big three: sleep, healthy eating and exercise.

Depression and Sleep

The connection between sleep and depression is huge. In fact, this is one of the primary areas in which current protocols for treating depression have to change dramatically, since what we know from current research just isn't often put into practice. Most therapy for depression focuses on medication or medication plus cognitive-behavioral therapy. Research is showing that sleep may actually be *causal* in depression and other mood disorders, but this idea hasn't permeated practice by a long shot. You must, must, change your life to get enough sleep if you want to have any hope of maintaining your psychological and physiological health.

Not only is poor sleep now considered a cause of depression, but poor sleep can also keep an already depressed person depressed[124]. To make matters worse, a previously depressed person is more likely to have worse sleep, even after depression has gone away. One study found that 45% of adults with previous (but not current) depression showed symptoms of troubled sleep as compared to just 17% of adults without previous depression.[125] Also, symptoms of continuing difficulties with sleep increase the risk that depression will return.[126]

Take a Look at Your Relationship with Sleep

If you aren't regularly sleeping around eight hours per night, it's important for you to take a close look at your relationship with sleep. Check out our points on how to get better control of your sleep found earlier in the book. If you are depressed, and having a lot of trouble with your sleep, please know that there are a number of things that will improve sleep even for a person with depression. But all of them involve doing something (like exercise), and when you are depressed, it's awfully hard to get yourself to do anything. Therefore, I recommend that you seek professional help, and perhaps additionally enlist a close friend to help you get started.

Depression and Social Support

The evidence that social support is tied to emotional well-being is very, very clear. What you may not have heard yet is that social support is also tied to physiological well-being. Being with people actually improves your immune system in a number of ways. T-cells and NK cells are important parts of your immune system. Both are influenced by being with people. Support groups for people struggling with cancer have become more of the norm today because of their observed positive effect on physiological as well as psychological functioning. Simply put, people who socialize more die slower. Having a reliable network of social support is an important priority for anyone – even introverted individuals who tend to spend less time and effort nurturing their social support network.

Depressed people tend to withdraw from social functioning. One of the therapies that helps with depression involves something called "Activation" therapy. The idea here is to get more active. Go out and do things, become more involved, be with people even when you don't want to be. And when you are depressed, sometimes you really, really don't want to be with people! Spending time socializing may seem overwhelming and it may seem like the last thing you are interested in when you are depressed. Much of getting better from depression depends on your willingness to do the things necessary to get better even when you really don't feel like it. There are no magic pills for anyone, and the "work" of getting better is definitely hard work.

Depression and Exercise

You simply cannot underestimate the impact of exercise on depression...or on any "mental" illness. I cannot stress enough that the impact of exercise on your overall health and emotional well-being is so pervasive that absolutely no one can afford to not exercise. I read a great quote by Edward Stanley the other day: "Those who think they have not time for BODILY EXERCISE will sooner or later have to find time for illness." Even psychiatric medical research supports exercise as a first-line treatment for depression; one study found that exercise was as effective as a particular antidepressant (specifically sertraline, also known as Zoloft) [127] Other research has found that people who use exercise to combat depression have lower relapse rates than people who were on antidepressants[128].

Exercise does far more than merely boost endorphins, make you feel good about yourself, or even create new brain cells. Exercise sets off a far-reaching network of positive effects on the brain, the body and your mood[129], a network of effects that is far beyond what I could tell you in this book. Simply put, exercise *is* brain health in action.

Depression and Nutrition

I go over the importance of nutrition with all my clients, depressed or not. For a long time science claimed that diet had little or no relationship to mental health. Some of these claims are rapidly falling by the wayside as investigators take a more careful and better instrumented look at the role of nutrition in mental disorders. Here's just one example: A recent study shows that depression is linked to plasma levels of carotenoids.[130] Carotenoids come from colorful vegetables and fruits like carrots, spinach, sweet potatoes, bell peppers, kale, tomatoes and papayas. In a sample of nearly 1000 older men and women (65 years old or more), higher blood levels of carotenoids were associated with a significantly lower likelihood of depressed mood six years later. Low levels of carotenoids predicted depression. So eating your vegetables, especially the colorful kind, will protect you from depression down the road.

Depression and Past History

Trauma happens to many of us, and perhaps to most of us. Some of us have experienced truly horrific events that are beyond what we consider "normal" life. Past trauma can leave its mark in the way we manage emotions, the way our brain looks or acts (physiological traces), and particularly in our learned behaviors (the way we perceive and react to various events). The good news is that we can change our lives enough to leave trauma in the past. We can teach our minds and bodies new and more adaptive responses for the happenings of the present moment. My primary emphasis in this area is to stress the following: If you are interested in change, you must create change with your whole self (body and mind). You must create mind-body health, without waiting another moment. Your brain was shaped by your past, but you can reshape it in your present based on how you care for it. You have a choice. You can give in to the past and give up on change, staying miserable. Or you can do everything necessary to effect real change. There are things you can do that will indeed work, and refusing to do them in order to more fully affix blame on something/someone else is only going to keep you miserable. Sure, you don't want to exercise. Sure, whatever happened was not your fault. But you are the one in the present moment who is living your life. So live your life, don't let your past live it for you! Your past will live it miserably. But you have all the power you need to decide to be courageous and live differently.

New Ideas About Depression

What we have seen so far is that science shows that depression is responsive to what we've traditionally thought of as exclusively physical things like probiotics, exercise, vitamin D, omega-3 fatty acids, and better quality sleep. What scientists have most recently uncovered is perhaps even more unexpected:

A growing body of evidence (including three meta-analyses[131]) shows that depression is compellingly linked to inflammation[132, 133, 134]. That is, not only is the number of previous depressive episodes associated with increased inflammation markers later, but also that inflammatory responses are also associated with the onset of depression as well as the risk of its recurrence.

One of the original clues to this link between depression and inflammation was that when patients were given the drug Interferon, which increases inflammation, they then had a high likelihood of developing symptoms (if not a diagnosable episode) of depression within a few months[135].

Some people with depression may have normal levels of inflammation, and some other people without depression may have high levels of inflammation. Yet the evidence shows that, as a group, people with depression generally have higher levels of inflammation than people without depression. Also, while the amount of increased inflammation that is associated with depression may be relatively minor, it is at the same time sufficient to create significant risk for developing later inflammation-related problems such as heart disease, stroke, cancer, diabetes and dementia[136]. The likely sticking point that prevents some from completely buying the inflammation-depression link is that inflammation is connected to so many other variables in addition to depression, that it is difficult to identify specific and reliable pathways to and from depression.

So if depression is linked to inflammation, of course my immediate thought is about all the "physical" treatments we've been talking about. I find it very compelling that the list of what helps reduce depression (exercise, vitamin D, omega-3 fatty acids, and sleep) are *all* things that reduce inflammation![137,138]

One thing really does lead to another, doesn't it?

Inflammation and Depression

If your physician has recently run any blood tests to search for markers of inflammation, one of those tests was likely a CRP level, which stands for C-Reactive Protein. CRP is just what it says it is: a protein found in the blood that reacts to your level of overall inflammation and can therefore be used as a measure of inflammation. Higher levels of CRP indicate higher general inflammation, which in turn indicates that there is a problem that must be solved. Just what the problem is, however, is less clear. Sometimes higher inflammation is linked with using hormone replacement therapy, or with obesity or even with pregnancy. Because CRP is a somewhat general indicator of inflammation levels, it doesn't point to any specific disease but instead shows you that there may be an underlying infection or inflammation in your body. Lower CRP levels are better for your risk of a number of inflammation related diseases, including heart disease. CRP levels are also related to depression. A 2012 article links CRP levels to cumulative episodes of depression, showing that in 1420 people (including children), the cumulative amount of depression for each person was significantly associated with CRP levels[139]. Depression also increases the risk of inflammation in heart failure patients, another inflammatory disease state[140]. So it looks like there is evidence for the idea that depression today can raise your level of inflammation tomorrow.

One Thing Multiplies Another Exponentially

A poor diet, concurrent with stress (stress can include depression) combine to create even worse conditions than either one would create on its own. A poor diet plus stress is not merely additive in its negative impact on depression. A part of the reason for that is that stress creates an even poorer metabolic response to unhealthy meals than you would normally have if you weren't depressed. Your food choices are important! They affect your moods in addition to affecting inflammation and the activity of the vagus nerve, the long nerve that extends from the brain throughout some of the body. And vagus nerve activity also turns around to affect inflammation. Here the effect is good: stimulating the vagus nerve can decrease inflammation. Stimulating the vagus nerve also helps relieve depression. The vagus nerve is also involved in the healthy digestion, absorption and metabolism of nutrients[141]...which in turn further influence inflammation, and depression. If you aren't already dizzy from reading this paragraph, you are seeing that the connections here are incredibly multilayered.

Here are yet more layers: your gut health is absolutely central to your overall level of inflammation. Not only is there a correlation between depression and gastrointestinal inflammation, but an increasing number of clinical studies point to the usefulness of probiotics, omega-3 fatty acids, vitamin D and the B vitamins in the treatment of inflammation for the body, for the brain, and for depression [142].

To sum up, inflammation and depression are inextricably related. Inflammation also appears to underlie a whole host of other disorders. As far as your health goes, it may be that inflammation is not just one of many risk factors – it may be that it is the one risk factor that underlies all the others.

At this point it should be clear to you that treating depression is best done by using the body in addition to the mind. Leaving the body out of any depression treatment plan simply goes against the empirical evidence. Understanding the pervasive impact of the body on depression can be incredibly hopeful to folks who struggle. Rather than relying on medication that may not be helpful, and comes with a number of unwanted side effects, you can have a great deal more power over your mental health by *Fix*ing your physiological health.

Holistic Context

One thing that's important to point out is that since one thing always leads to another, we must realize that there are a multiplicity of reasons that depression happens. A "one-pill fix" is unrealistic, as there is almost always more than one thing wrong. Relying on one intervention alone without looking at the overall context of the particular fix you are trying to make is like attempting to get your car to start when it's missing half the engine. Sure, it might be out of gas, but adding gas isn't going to be enough to fix the problem. And once the engine is fixed, it will still need gas. Similarly, some of the interventions that target depression are necessary but not sufficient on their own. If you continue to eat processed foods and drink sugar, taking a probiotic to fix your depression just won't be enough. This doesn't mean that probiotics don't work, it just means that you can't ignore the holistic context of your health and think that one targeted intervention will be enough to overcome everything else that's out of whack.

Where to Start Now?

Now that you read the material in this chapter, sit back for a few moments. Take a look at your life. Identify those factors that are actively contributing to how things are going for you. Ponder what you might be able to do differently. Then circle or list the top two or three things you feel most interested in tackling right now.

And especially, since this is the chapter

about depression, if you are, or think you may be, struggling with clinical depression right now, consult a professional.

Remember, it's okay to feel unmotivated. Feeling unmotivated has little to do with whether or not you actually put into practice helpful behaviors. You can take this list below to your doctor and ask for support in immediately implementing some of the elements of this plan.

An Evidence-Based Mind-Body Program to Treat Depression:

1. Try an adaptogen blend (see the sidebar) to help give yourself the strength and energy to begin treatment, and to begin to do some of the other things that feel just too overwhelming without a little boost. Also, many adaptogens have a mood-lifting effect and act to decrease depression and anxiety.

2. Add vitamin D3 (with K2) and a good quality omega-3 fatty acid supplement. Don't skimp on these – you need plenty of both. Remember, a therapeutic level is what you are aiming for.

> **What Are Adaptogens?**
> Adaptogens are a class of herbs that have a non-specific benefit to the body. They can improve the body's reactions to stress, boost energy, improve the immune system and improve mood and sleep among a number of other benefits. Some examples include:
> Rhodiola
> Eleuthero
> Astragalus
> American Ginseng
> Ashwagandha

3. Start exercising. Yes, if you are depressed, more effort is required to start exercising than if you were not depressed, so start slowly, because this step can feel pretty daunting. You might just try a little 2-minute bounce on a rebounder to begin with. Anything is better than nothing. Be gentle on your body so that you do not injure yourself, as this will set you back further than you want to be. Be smart so that you gradually increase what you are doing without overwhelming yourself.

4. Get in the sun, daily if you can, and spend a few minutes engaged in "sunning" yourself. This isn't about getting tan, it's about exposing yourself to the healing force of the sun. Stretch and breathe and soak in some of those great vitamin-D producing rays. Standing in the sun in the morning when you awaken will help your circadian rhythms. We also know that sun exposure increases serotonin levels. A therapeutic level is reached before your skin turns pink.

5. Fix the gut. This includes treating food allergies (or at least, not eating the foods that provoke allergies), treating "leaky gut" problems, reducing sugar intake (probably drastically), drinking water and eliminating sodas and fruit juices (not whole fruits), and taking a quality probiotic. Take that probiotic properly, which usually means that you take it without anything other than water, about 20 minutes before you eat.

6. Do something every day that gives you a sense of accomplishment. Do something that's a little bit challenging but not too overwhelming. I like to say that you are looking for a balance somewhere between the work involved in shutting and opening a door (way too easy) versus curing cancer (too hard). Do something daily that you can feel proud of, even if it's "just" cleaning your kitchen counters or changing the oil in your car. The important part of your decision here is not so much what you choose to do but that you allow yourself to *feel* the accomplishment! Don't crush your sense of accomplishment in a task completed by instantly telling yourself that it wasn't really that big of a deal, that anyone could do the same thing, or that you should have done it before now anyway! If every accomplishment is like a brick in the wall against depression, telling yourself that your accomplishments are no good is like employing your very own brick demolition machine. Making bricks just to crush them simply isn't a good use of energy! If you do find yourself thinking that your achievements are nothing to take joy in, just kindly notice that this is what you are doing, and then move gently away from that thought.

7. Fix distorted cognitions and increase your level of emotional regulation. One contributor to depression that may remain, even after many of the issues listed above have been largely taken care of, is an impoverished sense of self. Lack of healthy boundaries, lack of positive self-regard and a sense of general incompetence can all contribute to this sense of self-impoverishment. A common thread underlying each of these "lacks"

is one great big dearth of what, in psychology circles, has begun to be called "self-compassion." See the Self-Compassion chapter for more information.

8. Do something every day to boost your mood beyond those things that give you a sense of accomplishment. In addition to exercise, dancing and singing are also mood-lifting and healing to the brain's emotional systems. Looking at pictures of loved ones helps calm the brain. Another way to "wake up" your rational brain and calm feelings of anxiety is to play word games that involve finding common connections between different, random words. For example, one thought that might connect the words camel, bureau and hovercraft is this: "I leaped from the hovercraft onto a camel and strapped the bureau drawer behind me as we galloped off!" There are no right or wrong ways to connect words. You can connect them with a story, or through things you notice about the letters or syllables. Really, any connecting idea will create the kind of brain impact you are looking for. Finding a connecting idea about seemingly unrelated objects boosts endorphins and results in positive mood[143]. Purposely add daily activities that will bring you pleasant feelings. You have to plan to go get these feelings – you can't wait for them to drop on you out of the sky. It's normal to have to plan in order to make these kinds of things happen. If you are stuck thinking that regular people automatically experience mood-boosting events without even having to plan them, take some time to challenge this distorted thought.

9. Try adding things like light therapy or cranial electrotherapy stimulation (see alpha-stim.com). Both of these interventions are very useful clinically and both have good bases in science. Data show that Alpha-Stim treatment out-performs antidepressants, is anti-inflammatory, helps you sleep better and reduces anxiety.

10. Be gentle with yourself. Trying to force yourself out of depression is not effective in the long term and it often doesn't work in the short term either. Doing the things we've listed will help your mood eventually. Worrying about being depressed will only make things worse. Go easy. Just take it one step at a time...preferably a step outside in the sun and with your walking shoes on!

Chapter Thirteen

Irritable Bowel Syndrome

Nearly everyone remembers hearing the phrase "you are what you eat." Ad nauseam, right? The truth of it is that you are what you eat more than you or your fifth grade science teacher could ever have suspected.

First of all, you're only one-tenth human. Perhaps your siblings or spouse have told you this already!

But all kidding aside, your body is mostly bacteria, in fact, bacteria outnumber human cells 10 to 1. This number isn't about size or weight, as bacteria are much smaller than human cells. We carry inside us a tremendous number of amazing bacteria (friendly flora) that we absolutely rely on to function. It may be that nowhere in the body this is more true than in your gut.

If you really understood all the great things that your gut bacteria did for you, you'd be taking very good care of them and thanking them morning, noon and night. Perhaps this chapter will inspire you to do some of that thanking by paying careful attention to what you eat morning, noon and night. What you eat has a powerful effect on gut bacteria, and as you'll see, gut bacteria is the foundation of digestive health. In fact, leading scientists in the field now theorize that an imbalance in digestive flora is perhaps the primary cause of Irritable Bowel Syndrome.

IBS is an excellent example of a problem with multiple causes and multiple solutions. One of the reasons for this confusion surrounding IBS is that people are frantically trying to identify the Magic Bullet answer — the one thing that caused it and the one thing that will cure it. The result of this frenzied search and discard mission is that it's easy to miss the big picture when you're looking for a Magic Bullet.

When I was in graduate school, I never dreamed bowel functioning might be related to things like depression, or that so many[ww] of my anxious clients would also have digestive trouble. I also never imagined that teaching clients how

---

[ww] My clients think I'm magically divining reality when I ask about their digestive trouble. Until I tell them, they don't realize that pretty much every single anxious client I see also has significant stomach problems.

their gut functioned would be a relevant part of psychologically oriented therapy! But bowel health is crucially, foundationally important.

What is Irritable Bowel Syndrome (IBS)?

Irritable bowel syndrome (IBS) is a term for a group of problems primarily involving abdominal pain, abdominal bloating and constipation and/or diarrhea. Until recently, medical science believed that IBS had no physical cause and was simply the result of patients' becoming distressed about the functioning of their bowels. They were prescribed this or that medication (usually laxatives or anti-diarrhea drugs) and then shoved off on their merry way. But now physicians are starting to realize that IBS is a real disorder with physical causes. Nonetheless, the science underlying our understanding of IBS remains limited by what we can measure.

> **What is the Gut?**
> The term "gut" refers to any of the following: the gastrointestinal tract, the digestive tract, the GI tract, the alimentary canal, and sometimes the stomach and intestines. Gut is a term used both throughout the medical and scientific literature as well as outside the medical literature.

What we do know is this: The most common symptoms of IBS are abdominal pain, the relief of that abdominal pain with bowel action, passing mucous through the bowels and a feeling of incomplete evacuation. IBS typically flares up now and again and then it seems to go into remission. The average symptom flare-ups last about seven days per month with two bouts per day (lasting on average an hour each). Flare-ups are often associated with stress such as anxiety or depression,[144] and some theorize that because of the mind-gut connection, flare-ups even cause anxiety and depression.

IBS is a very common problem and it's actually the second-most common reason people miss work, right after the common cold. At least 10-15% of the general population suffers from IBS,[145] with some population estimates reaching as high as 20%.[146]

IBS occurs more frequently in women than in men. The most common conventional treatments involve symptom management through either medication or lifestyle changes (things like eliminating dairy products or increasing exercise).

When initially diagnosed with IBS, many people receive the discouraging news from their doctors that they may be stuck with this misery for the rest of their lives. But data actually show that half of all IBS patients have recovered by their next follow-up visit. Also, resolving stressors (divorce, bankruptcy, etc.) helps some people with IBS to significantly improve,[147] because the mind-body connection works both ways. It can help set off illness and it can also help resolve illness.

You can imagine that, during a bout of IBS, the affected person might be thinking "Why, oh why me?" as IBS sounds dreadfully miserable. Recent developments in science are indeed working on the question of "Why anyone?" As the connection between brain and gut becomes more apparent in study after study, it is easier to see how major stressors (mind) can impact the immune system (body). This connection is yet another clear example of why continuing to believe in the mind-body split is so last-century. Now let's dive further into the details.

Many Causal Contributors

There are a large number of hypothesized contributors to the development of IBS. Some of these contributors simply create a vulnerability and others are favored as potential underlying causes of IBS. One of the reasons there is so much confusion in this area is, like I said, that researchers are looking for *the* cause: the Magic Bullet. What I detail here are some of the multiple possibilities that likely contribute. Rather than one single magic cause, IBS is probably just like that Mustang with the mass airflow sensor problem that I mentioned back in the second chapter. The fix requires multiple solutions for multiple causes.

Family History & Social Learning

Having a family history of the problem is a risk factor. This is because genetics contribute to IBS as well as the things you learn from your family through social interaction ("social learning"). These socially learned factors can include everything from bolting your food without chewing to staying up late because of severe anxiety.

Prior Infection, Food Allergies and Gluten

Prior bacterial or viral stomach infections also strongly increase your risk of IBS. Gastroenteritis increases the risk of IBS by seven-fold. Food allergies, Candida overgrowth and gluten intolerance all have the potential to damage epithelial gut tissue, thereby creating vulnerability to infection by pathogens. A tremendous amount of information (albeit confusing and contradictory) is easily available about these topics and it would probably take several books to properly discuss these issues. So I will leave it to you to investigate further if you are interested.

Stress and IBS

Perhaps none of the diseases we've talked about in this book are blamed on stress as often as irritable bowel syndrome. There's a good reason for this fact — people who are under stress really are much more likely to have symptoms of IBS. For instance, a study of over 1700 nursing and medical students (people who we know are stressed out!) showed that their rate of IBS was double or triple the rate of IBS in the general population[148]. Not only that, but over 40% of the females in this group of high-stress students suffered from IBS. Those that had IBS also had significantly higher anxiety, depression, stressful life events, and sleeping disorders. Interestingly, they also spent more time sitting rather than standing or walking compared to the other people in the study, and they missed more meals and ate more processed foods.

Some studies suggest that the kind of stress we're talking about here is "big" stress — the kind related to clinical anxiety and depression, and not the ordinary kind that comes from daily, more run-of-the-mill stressors[149]. One study suggested that it may be that for women, clinical anxiety and depression are what predict

IBS symptoms, but for men, work-related stress is what brings on IBS[150].

Evidence strongly points to stress both as a significant contributor to IBS flare-ups as well as to the constancy and severity of IBS symptoms[151]. One explanation for this is cortisol, the hormone released when a person experiences stress. When cortisol release is signaled during stress, gastrointestinal functioning changes. This change stimulates the immune system to release pro-inflammatory cells that can create low-grade inflammation in the gut. In most of the population, cortisol helps reduce this kind of inflammation but in IBS patients, levels of proinflammatory cells remain high[152]. When your body constantly reacts to stressors as if you're being chased by a tiger, it's likely that either your stress response is a problem or that there are a LOT of tigers around. The interaction between stress responses and the immune system seems to be what makes IBS symptoms worse.

History of Abuse and IBS

In addition to current life stressors such as work or school, stressors like childhood or adult abuse also increase the likelihood of IBS.[153]

Specifically, women with IBS are more likely to have experienced physical punishment, emotional or sexual abuse or general trauma in their past. Of those factors, the strongest predictor of IBS was emotional abuse[154] — a good reason to seek competent help in recovering from any kind of abuse, including emotional abuse.

Schizandra: An Adaptogen

Schisandra chinensis, commonly known as schizandra, is a berry plant native to China. In fact, its Chinese name comes from the fact that its berries seem to possess all five of the basic flavors (sweet, salty, sour, spicy and bitter). So it's definitely not the kind of berry you pop in your mouth or make into pie. It's medicinal, and it tastes like it.

Schizandra is known for far more than its taste, however. It's one of the most important herbs in Traditional Chinese Medicine, indicating that it has been used over and over for more than 2,000 years.

The berry is known for increasing energy, boosting the immune system and its protective effect on organs such as the liver, the kidneys and the lungs. It also has been shown to improve concentration, endurance, accuracy and mood.

As an adaptogen, schizandra has an overall beneficial effect on the body. It helps at the cellular level, providing nutrients, anti-oxidants and anti-inflammatory action to heal and support nourishment.

Early Stress & Increased Gut Pain Sensitivity

There is some evidence that early life stressors affect what's called the "visceral sensitivity" (sensitivity to pain) of the gut. This research was done using an animal model of pain and stress. Rats were stressed by being separated from their mothers at an early age. When compared to rats who were not stressed in this way, the stressed rats had higher gut pain. Interestingly, the rats in this study were then given the adaptogenic herb *schizandra*. Those who received schizandra showed an increase in their pain threshold. The study concluded that schizandra can reverse visceral sensitivity in the gut (at least in rats).[155]

SIBO: A Serious Causal Contender

SIBO[xx] (Small Intestine Bacterial Overgrowth) is thought of as a clear contributor to IBS although it's a problem we are still learning about. We think SIBO occurs when the small intestine suffers from an overgrowth of bacteria. It may be this infection happens when there are not enough friendly flora to kill off invading pathogens, so they get to the small intestine and multiply. We aren't really certain yet because we don't understand the small intestine well enough.

In order to explain, let me help you with a little "geography" first. The stomach connects to the small intestine, of which there are three parts. The part right where it connects to the stomach is called the *duodenum*. The long middle part is called the *jejunum;* it's about one inch in diameter and about 8 feet long. The last part of the small intestine is the *ileum*, and it's between 6-13 feet long. The place where the large intestine hooks up to the small intestine is called the *cecum*. The large intestine, or colon, climbs up from your lower right side, goes across your

---

[xx] Not the place in Sweden! You can still travel to Sweden without damaging your small intestine.

middle and down your left side into the rectum, eventually ending at the opening called the anus. The large intestine is about three inches in diameter.

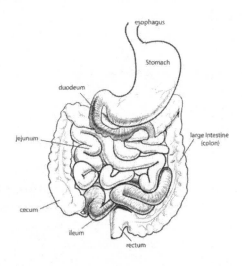

Food is broken down first in your mouth and then in your stomach into a gooey substance called *chyme.* Chyme travels into the small intestine where any available nutrition is taken into the body as much as possible. The large intestine can extract some nutrition as well, but its primary purpose is to extract water from the chyme, turning it into stool so that the waste can exit the body. Once the stool enters the rectum there is a feeling of urgency to evacuate the bowel. Although it's normal for stool to be in the colon, the rectum should ordinarily be empty. Stool that is not completely evacuated from the rectum dries up, creating blockage.

One theory about the cause of IBS is that bacteria somehow find a passage through the cecum back into the small intestine (backwards through the *ileocecal* valve), and then these bacteria wreak all kinds of havoc in the small intestine. Thus, when IBS responds well to antibiotics, as it occasionally does, this positive response is possibly because those pathogenic bacteria in the small intestine are finally being killed off. But afterward, since the original problem — the gateway that allows bacteria to travel from the large to the small intestine — remains open, bacteria eventually climb up into the small intestine again, setting off another round of IBS flare-ups. Then, thanks to the previous antibiotic treatment, the probiotic population that might have helped keep pathogens under control is now no longer able to function nearly as well. This is just one explanation for how SIBO may contribute to IBS. At this point, scientists just don't have enough information yet to form clearer answers.

Motility: Another Causal Factor

A related theory deals with what's called *motility,* meaning the coordinated motion of the intestines.[156] After you eat, your intestines regularly contract and move food, or *chyme,* back and forth along their passageways, mixing it with digestive enzymes. The food then moves through the small intestine and into the large intestine. This can take between two and five hours. When you haven't eaten, your small intestines have a different pattern of movement that is nonetheless important. About every 90 minutes they contract, acting to sweep any remaining food particles toward the large intestine.[157] Intestines move in waves. Motility is connected to IBS in at least two ways. First, these movements can cause pain due to overactive nerves in the gut. Alternatively, lack of motility creates opportunity for bacteria overgrowth, and may lead to SIBO. Factors that can decrease motility include lack of sleep, lack of exercise, avoiding going to the bathroom and emotional distress.

Inflammation: A Central Causal Factor

Finally, low-grade inflammation is a clear overall contributor to IBS.[158] In fact, one emerging hypothesis is that low-grade inflammation is central to what goes wrong when a person has IBS[159]. The effect on IBS of "leaky gut," or the gut permeability process (which we discussed in the chapter about inflammation) is a cutting-edge theory for understanding IBS. Leaky gut is what results when food particles and bacteria escape the stomach and GI tract through small spaces created by damaged intestinal lining. Damaged lining can result from inflammation, irritants like medications[yy], sugar, food allergies or stress chemicals, etc. In turn, leaky gut increases general inflammation. Many people link leaky gut to the onset of IBS symptoms.

Inflammation and the Gut Biome

In this chapter we continue to see that healthy gut bacteria are absolutely critical to overall health. As discussed so far in this book, a problematic gut biome is associated with

---

[yy] Even birth control pills can create these kinds of irritations; birth control pills also kill probiotics.

inflammation, heart disease[160], depression, and diabetes[zz]. IBS is even more closely grounded in the gut than these other conditions.

Stop for a moment and take a look at your gut bacteria history. How many times did you take antibiotics? Antibiotics can be incredibly useful in certain circum-stances, but they all have the side effect of destroying friendly flora as well as pathogens. How many pharmaceutical medications have you taken? Most medications irritate the mucosal lining of the gut, and kill probiotics as well. What about cholorinated or fluoridated water? Both chlorinated and fluoridated water kill friendly flora. Junk food? Sugar? Yes, they kill probiotics too. Sugar in particular can be problematic because sugar feeds bad bacteria which in turn can kill good bacteria. Even if you are more healthy and careful than the typical American, your gut has likely suffered some impacts from these substances common in modern-day life.

> *One emerging hypothesis is that low-grade inflammation is central to what goes wrong when a person has IBS*

Medical scientists know that antibiotics will kill at least some of the probiotics residing inside you. Traditionally this has been passed off as a minimal problem. But we now know that antibiotic use can change the gut biome permanently![161] Not only are we left much more

---

[zz] It's also a major player in asthma and allergies.

vulnerable to a host of disease-promoting organisms when we don't have our friendly flora to protect us, but we also have more trouble rebuilding a population that contains primarily healthy bacteria. As mentioned in the inflammation chapter, unfriendly flora can be pro-inflammatory; when these kinds of flora have a strong presence in the gut, the overall action of the biome changes.

Your gut has a long history, starting as you were born. Newborns receive their first dose of healthy bacteria when they travel down the birth canal. Children born by C-section do not have this benefit and their gut flora suffers accordingly. Even when children are born vaginally, they are still affected by antibiotics the mother may have taken during pregnancy as well as the amount of sugar in their newborn diets. Commercial baby foods and formula are among the culprits; babies fed formula have vastly different gut biomes from breastfed babies.[162] And the early assault on the gut biome doesn't stop there, by any means. The average child receives about 20 courses of antibiotics by the time he or she reaches adulthood. Science is just beginning to link this kind of long-term exposure to antibiotics to increased incidence of allergies, asthma, obesity and metabolic disorders as well as to inflammatory bowel diseases.[163]

As I read this research, I kind of took it personally. When pregnant with my daughter I had been diagnosed with Lyme disease, and was given antibiotics. This same daughter struggles with relatively severe asthma and allergies. Now it's important to note that her father also has asthma and allergies, and we know there are genetic contributions as well as environmental contributions to both asthma and allergies. This example from my own family further supports my belief that our mind-body health exists in a context wherein there are multiple causes and multiple effects. There is no Magic Bullet either in cause or solution.

Some of us used to not worry much about taking antibiotics as it was assumed that simply taking probiotics would easily restore the friendly flora right back to its former glory. But what current research reveals is that it's not so simple. Antibiotic use appears to permanently change the gut biome, both in overall numbers of probiotics and in the number of kinds (strains). Taking probiotics doesn't seem to be a strong enough treatment to fully counter the impact of antibiotic use. This solution is on the right track, but it doesn't go far enough.

When I consider this problem, I think of the following things: First, since taking probiotics to counter antibiotics is clearly a Magic Bullet solution, I'm not surprised that it doesn't entirely fix the problem. Second, our ancestors didn't use pills to build their probiotic population! They ate garden vegetables with soil traces on them, whereas we scrub our vegetables clean of any trace of dirt. Soil contains a multitude of bacteria[aaa] and our

> *Studies find that after antibiotics the friendly flora never fully recover.*

[aaa] Soil bacteria is where two common antibiotics were discovered: streptomycin and neomycin.

ancestors have been ingesting it for millennia. Our ancestors also used a number of fermented foods in their diets, and such foods are marvelous sources of probiotics. The average American eats virtually no fermented foods[bbb]. (No, beer doesn't count! Alcohol kills probiotics. And grocery store yogurts hardly resemble real, fermented yogurt. Plus, the added sugars kill probiotics by feeding other microbes like Candida.) There is a real problem here, and this problem requires a holistic solution, not a Magic Bullet wherein you simply pop a probiotic pill and think you are home free.

The Brain-Gut Axis

Research tells us that the balance between good and harmful gut bacteria plays a role not only in gut functioning, but also in brain functioning. That is to say, disruptions in gut bacteria can disturb what's called the brain-gut axis[164]. Simply put, the "brain-gut axis" is the connection between brain functioning (nerves, sensations, etc.) and intestinal muscle tightening, pain sensations and so forth. Things that affect the brain, for instance depression or anxiety, also affect the gut and vice-versa: things that affect the gut also affect the brain. This is why my patients with anxiety also struggled with recurrent stomach problems.

The difference between IBS and some of the other problems discussed in this book is that IBS, is by conventional definition, *not* due to any

---

[bbb] Take a look at the sourdough breads at your grocer. Most of them contain yeast.

underlying diagnosed medical problem, and is seen by conventional medicine primarily as a mind-body disease[ccc]. For example, a doctor is likely to view IBS as a result of chronic anxiety rather than as a physiologically based disease that can be exacerbated by psychological symptoms. I've had many patients who were told that IBS was all in their heads, and they just needed to be less anxious. However the data clearly show that IBS is not "all in your head." If your doctor tells you it is, go find someone who is willing to work harder to get a better answer. Once you solve the problem of not being taken seriously —because, believe me, it's not just in your head!— you can take comfort in knowing that you can find relief through paying attention to primarily physiological principles of good bowel functioning. Of course, we won't ignore helping you learn how to reduce anxiety and resolve stressors. Your decisions to change how you eat, your new sleep practices, exercise habits, your improved ways of managing stress and your healthier bowel habits will all affect your gut health and can create a wonderful healing environment for IBS.

IBS and Exercise

When people with IBS increase their levels of physical activity, they experience fewer symptoms. Exercising three to five times per week results in significant improvement. People with IBS who do not increase exercise actually

---

[ccc] Ever notice how gas stations are chock-full of anti-diarrhea medicine and laxatives? "Houston? Houston?"

experience more symptoms than they might have had they started exercising. That is to say, symptoms worsen significantly less over time with physical activity than without.[165] In addition to preventing worsening symptoms, exercise can specifically help decrease the painful symptoms of constipation.[166] Moving the body helps move the bowels (motility!), and moving the bowels is primary to good gut health!

Exercise will improve digestion in people whether or not they have IBS. Here's a fun word: post-prandial; it means after a meal. Post-prandial exercise would include a walk after dinner. Walking after a meal (not sprinting) can be a nice way to improve digestion. You will be taking good care of your gut biome, as well as reducing stress, which is also good for your gut.

IBS and Sleep

Generally, people with IBS also have poor sleep, and this is another chicken-egg quandary. Which comes first – poor sleep or IBS? The connection between poor sleep and IBS is found in young people. Asian teens who sleep poorly are twice as likely to have IBS than their peers who sleep well.[167] The same is true for adults: The worse sleep you have, the worse your IBS symptoms.[168]

Researchers have found that IBS patients who also have problematic sleep also have a lower threshold for urges to move their bowels. They experience more bowel pain when compared to IBS patients who don't have sleep problems[169]. So poor sleep makes things worse all around.[ddd]

[ddd] Not only does poor sleep make it harder to have a good enough

This sleep-IBS connection gets even more interesting when you factor in circadian rhythm. Circadian rhythm is your body's daily activity cycle, as was discussed in the Sleep chapter. Circadian rhythms influence digestive processes[170]. The gastrointestinal tract itself actually keeps a circadian rhythm that is responsible for all of the regular movement in your gut muscles (muscle waves from your stomach to your colon). Disruptions to this circadian rhythm, which can be caused by things like difficulty sleeping or shift work, can create such trouble in the gut that these disruptions can actually set off problems like IBS[171].

IBS and Diet: A Controversial Mess!

Reports of dietary influences on IBS are controversial in the scientific literature. Although dairy is often implicated clinically, there is little support for dairy actually being a contributor to IBS in the scientific literature.[172] But in the case of dairy, researchers have primarily examined the connection between IBS and lactose (milk sugar), and not between IBS and casein (milk protein). Researchers who think that lactic acid is a sufficient test of the impact of dairy on IBS symptoms will most likely extract that nutrient and use it alone in the study. After all, looking at only one potentially causal variable makes the overall research study more powerful. However, this approach then excludes other dairy factors

---

attitude to tolerate things that are a pain in the butt, but you actually feel more pain...

FODMAPS Diet

Researchers Peter Gibson and Susan Shepherd have developed the FODMAPS diet to treat IBS. FODMAPS is an acronym for Fermentable, Oligo-, Di-, Mono-saccharides and Polyols.

This diet restricts foods that contain fructans (these include but are not limited to wheat, onions, broccoli, cabbage, and chocolate), galactans (legumes are an example), polyols (apples, blackberries, peaches, watermelon, mushrooms, and sugars like xylitol, mannitol, and some others) and limits milk sugar (lactose) and fruit sugar (fructose).

Don't despair even though it looks like there's nothing left to eat. On the FODMAPS diet you can still eat blueberries, green beans, potatoes and meats among many other foods.

---

that may also impact IBS!

Although research doesn't support the idea that diet is reliably connected to IBS symptoms, most people with IBS attribute their symptoms to diet. Some of the common culprits identified by patients are thought to be vegetables (34%), fruit (29%), milk (15%), fat (15%), peppers and spices (6%) and sugar (4%).[173] This pretty much covers every kind of food but meat!

It's important to realize that it's hard to single out any individual foods as causing the worsening of IBS symptoms if they are eaten in the context of a traditional American diet and its already devastating impact on gut health. The likely reason research studies don't find a reliable connection between diet and IBS is due to the pre-existing context of most Americans'

Paleo Diet

Another diet many people with gut problems have found solace in is the Paleo diet, developed by Dr. Loren Cordain. Cordain uses interdisciplinary science to combine modern nutritional research with research done by anthropologists about living and dead hunter-gatherer cultures, their diets, and their rates of disease. He named his solution the Paleo diet because of the continuity he saw with the diet of our ancestors from the Paleolithic era, a 2.5 million year time period that ended about 10,000 years ago with the advent of agriculture. He argues that the agricultural revolution significantly changed the human diet.

Some people with IBS who follow the Paleo diet report improved symptoms and better health.

---

current proinflammatory diet.

There are a number of diets that people with IBS find useful. FODMAPS and Paleo diets are mentioned in sidebars but the GAPS and SCD diets can also be helpful. The fundamental similarity between these diets is a radical exclusion of all processed foods, flour and sugar, all of which damage the gut biome.

Sometimes doctors will prescribe an "exclusion" diet such that patients will eliminate foods such as milk, wheat and eggs. These types of exclusion diets vary in their effects on IBS, with some studies reporting a high percentage of improvement, and others reporting as low as only 15% improvement.[174]

The wide range of improvement results may, once again, rest on limitations in what researchers select to measure outcomes. For example, some research focuses on the amount of digestive gas as the main measure of IBS problems, and passes over other common symptoms of IBS. Other problems in the structuring and designing of IBS research studies include dividing people into different groups based on categorical criteria, when it is more likely that IBS, like most disease states, lies on a continuum.

Here's an example of problems in designing research studies. Celiac disease causes people to be unable to digest gluten. For these patients, dietary gluten causes significant problems in their bodies, usually resulting in IBS symptoms among other problems. Some people who do not meet the benchmark for a formal, clinical diagnosis of celiac disease may nonetheless have significant trouble digesting gluten. Consequently, these people may find clear improvement in their IBS symptoms when they eliminate gluten. The fact that digestive disorders like celiac exist on a continuum can create problems when researchers treat celiac disease as if it were categorical. For example, imagine that researchers ask volunteers to be a part of their study looking at the effect of a gluten-free diet on stomach pain. They then divide volunteers for the study into two categories as follows: 1) Patients with a celiac disease diagnosis, and 2) Patients without a celiac disease diagnosis. But since the patient groupings don't accurately represent real differences between the groups (because celiac is on a continuum), the effects of the treatment will be artificially diluted. Here's how: let's say a participant in the non-celiac group reports significantly less stomach pain on a gluten-free diet. A person in the celiac group also reports less pain. The gluten-free diet doesn't result in a big difference between the two groups' benefits. The power of the gluten-free diet to make a difference is therefore diluted because both groups benefit — not because the gluten-free diet doesn't have value. This example is about treatment dilution, but there are other kinds of research designs that result in faulty conclusions as well. Perhaps more often than we realize, so-called scientific research doesn't always do a good job of figuring out which treatments are useful. One of the lessons that we, the public, can learn from these problems is that simply because a study was performed doesn't meant that the study was designed well. Poor design means that the study conclusions may not be reliable. Poor design can happen when either the scientific method is not fully understood, or when it is not applied very well, but methodological design problems are definitely not an indication that science itself doesn't "work" or should be ignored!

Meat Controversy

Eating meat reduces friendly flora. Studies show that people who eat a vegan diet have different gut bacteria compared to those who are not vegan.[175] Eating meat also raises your risk of cancers. In fact, over 90% of gastrointestinal cancers are caused by environmental influences such as diet[176] so taking care of your gut flora can have a big impact! One study looked at diet, gut flora and colon cancer outcomes in three groups of people with different diets: Native

Africans, Caucasian Africans and African-Americans. The study was conducted to find out why West Africans had such a lower rate of colon cancer compared to the other groups. Among the three groups studied, Native Africans had indeed the lowest rate of colon cancer. The researchers attributed this to their diet. Native West Africans ate significantly less meat and other animal products, and much of their diet contained high fiber, starchy, spicy and peppery foods. [177] But there were two other factors in this study which I found most interesting: First, Native Africans had a lower dietary intake of what we consider to be important protective nutrients (vitamins C, A and E and calcium). Apparently eating animal fat and protein was such a powerful determinant of colon cancer risk that it far outweighed the relative risk of consuming significantly fewer protective nutrients. Second, there were clear differences in gut biome between the Native Africans and the other two groups[178]. Researchers explained that the impact of the foods eaten by Native Africans resulted in higher levels of protection in the colon due to the influence of the gut bacteria. Indeed, there seems to be a combination effect between gut biome and diet such that eating some foods in the presence of certain gut bacteria leads to higher risk of cancer as opposed to eating the same foods in the presence of different gut bacteria.[179]

On the other hand, meat eating (bone broth in particular) is strongly advocated as gut healing by a number of communities that address IBS symptoms. In particular, the Paleo community recommends meats as prime among healthful foods.

Healing IBS

There are a number of conventional treatments offered for people with IBS. Perhaps the most popular include fiber (bulking agents), antispasmodics, and antidepressants. But a Cochrane database review analyzed results from 56 randomized controlled trials comparing these three treatments with a placebo in patients diagnosed with IBS, and results showed no beneficial effect of bulking agents, (whether soluble or insoluble fiber). A small benefit was shown for antispasmodics[eee] in terms of reduced pain, but that benefit registered only about 12% better than placebo. Some pain reduction was also observed for patients who used antidepressants (20% over placebo)[180]. But when applied to children and adolescents with IBS, antidepressants showed no benefit[181].

These above treatments, fiber, antispasmodics and antidepressants, are clearly Magic Bullet style treatments. Simply examining the variable effects of fiber can demonstrate the complexity involved in IBS.

Fiber can be helpful for some but not helpful for others. The reasons underlying fiber's variable effectiveness depends on a multitude of individual differences in terms of what is actually going on in the gut of any individual with IBS. In some cases, the person with IBS is so constipated that adding additional fiber is more harmful than helpful.

[eee] cimteropium/ dicyclomine, peppermint oil, pinaverium and trimebutine

So adding more fiber is not only not always a useful approach for healing, but it can sometimes do more harm than good. Those Magic Bullets are not so magic after all.

The conventional, allopathic treatment of IBS in much of our world manages symptoms, not causes. Pain is a great example of a symptom and not a cause. Pain is a signal that something is wrong. Ignoring pain is like ignoring a traffic light by just closing your eyes and going straight on through! Yes, pain needs to be addressed, but it is the bowel function that needs to be restored. For this restoration, the bowel itself needs some healing.

An alternative approach to healing IBS may be found in the modality called Functional Medicine, an approach which focuses on treating and resolving underlying problems rather than merely relieving symptoms. The functional medicine approach to irritable bowel syndrome would be restoring proper bowel function rather than merely giving antidepressants or other medications to relieve pain. There are several ways to tackle improving bowel function, including restoring levels of helpful gut bacteria (probiotics), healing the stomach lining, and reducing psychological distress.

Probiotic pills (capsules that contain millions of helpful gut-directed bacteria) can help restore gut bacteria to higher levels of functioning, as long as dietary choices don't counteract their effects. Research finds that probiotic treatment significantly improves abdominal pain, diarrhea, bloating, and quality of life. Probiotic use in one study decreased the number of symptomatic days after only 1 month of treatment.[182] Both adults and children with IBS showed these benefits from probiotics.[183] When you consider purchasing probiotic supplements, select ones that contain both Lactobacillus and Bifidobacterium cultures, and choose ones with a variety of strains. Remember that simply taking probiotics is likely not a strong enough intervention so be sure to include a variety of fermented foods in your diet, too.

A number of studies also showed psycho-therapy or relaxation therapy to be helpful for improving IBS.[184] In order to achieve maximum benefit from psychotherapy, it is my recommen-dation that you do it while also working on improving sleep, exercise and diet.

Finally, there are a few other treatments that are worth a look. Capsaicin (found in spicy peppers and to a significantly lesser amount in bell peppers as well as in cumin and turmeric) is often helpful in treating pain and inflammation. One study found that capsaicin helped decrease abdominal pain and bloating in patients with IBS[185]. Artichoke leaf extract also shows promise as a substance to help reduce IBS symptoms[186]. The use of peppermint is relatively well known as way of relaxing the gastrointestinal tract, de-creasing pain, and adjusting immune system reactions[187]. Omega-3 fatty acids reduce inflam-mation throughout the body as well as in the gut[188], and finally, L-glutamine is an amino acid that can reverse leaky gut problems through its effects on gut tissue regeneration.[189]

Work to heal your gut lining rather than concentrate solely on managing symptoms. Change the materials your bowel is working with by eliminating as much processed food as you can. Increase exercise and sleep quality and reduce stress. For stress reduction — read on!

Chapter Fourteen

Self-Compassion

Gaille walked into my office feeling beat up by life. Prone to too much guilt and struggling against anxiety and depression, she just felt like she could never become the person she "should" have been already. She told me she couldn't reliably keep commitments to herself or her family. She became visibly uncomfortable when talking about letting someone down "yet again," and it was painful to hear her bitter self-criticism.

When Gaille came to treatment, she had asked for help in learning how to actually *do* what she already knew she needed to do. But what she really needed most was self-compassion. Here's an analogy: If Gaille were a building project under construction, self-compassion would be the needed rebar in her foundation.

Gaille wasn't raised to be kind to herself. Her parents were hard on themselves and they had high expectations of her. She agreed with those expectations, and contrary to popular magazine "wisdom," the solution to her self-described failure wasn't to change what she wanted of herself by lowering expectations. Rather, the solution was to strengthen her so she could become capable to reach higher. Previously, every time she stretched, she would sink a little farther. Firming up her foundation was the first step in helping Gaille achieve her goals.

Rather than first toning down depression and anxiety, Gaille's therapy began by cultivating positive emotions. Foremost was self-compassion, an emotion that has been shown to reduce the negative impacts of stress-induced cortisol and increase the soothing power that comes from relaxation-inducing hormones such as oxytocin. Self-compassion is a relatively new therapeutic component that has received a fair amount of attention in England, thanks to the work of Paul Gilbert. It has received a lesser amount of attention here in the United States, despite the valuable work of researchers such as Kristin Neff at UT-Austin.

Like many women (and women tend to struggle with self-compassion more than men), Gaille responded in three ways that are typical of people who are low in self-compassion behaviors:

1. She criticized herself, in some cases harshly and incessantly.
2. She increased her sense of isolation, by thinking "Nobody else is this bad" or "I don't deserve these friends."

3. She was stuck in a cycle of endless ruminating (worrying).

In fact, Gaille would often lie awake in bed, going over and over the problems she saw in herself, and feeling awful about her apparent inability to just "get over herself" and make positive changes. The shame, guilt, disappointment and anger she felt not only reduced her ability to be kind to others, but was also destroying her health. It was not surprising that she had trouble with irritable bowel syndrome, or that her frequent colds interfered with her work and attempts at exercise.

Suffering is Not Compassionate

Suffering is hard. We all do too much of it. Some of us were taught to suffer by parents or grandparents who were simply doing their best. But this legacy not only can be emotionally crippling, it can also get in the way of our achieving long-term growth and goals.

Over the past several decades, we have jumped on the hope that improving "self-esteem" was the answer to an impoverished sense of self. We prop up our self-disregard with affirmations, we create artificial successes so our children will feel good about themselves, and at the end of the day we still feel empty.

This is because, in our emotional suffering, we are facing a spiritual problem, not a success problem. Part of this problem is that we do not understand what it even means to treat ourselves with compassion, let alone know how to go about doing it. All the affirmations in the world won't fix a lack of self-compassion. And all the "self-esteem" in the world won't help you when you are faced with repeated discouragement and you are unable to find the motivation to do what you know would help you.

The key is simply this: the way to get yourself to do what you need to do isn't to beat yourself harder. Rather it's to learn to be self-compassionate.

Now before you jump to conclusions about what that actually means, let's talk about a few things that self-compassion *isn't*.

Self-Compassion: Not Self-Indulgence.

This is probably the most common misunderstanding about self-compassion that I run into. If you increase your level of self-compassion, you won't be in danger of ditching work, eating chocolate cake and watching "The Price is Right" all day. That's self-indulgence (well, self-indulgence for some, punishment for others!).

Self-Compassion: Not Entitlement or Self-pity.

Ever notice how we often tend to say "When things get back to normal..."? What is "normal" anyway? When I take a look at my life, the elusive "normal" doesn't happen often enough to technically qualify it as "normal!" Instead, I find myself in the midst of challenges and frustrations every day. And when I really take a moment to think about it, I prefer it this way. Life has a lot to teach me, and I'm not going to learn it sitting by the pool while someone else fills my drink!

We're all in the same boat. The times in our lives that are filled with peace and prosperity, love and success, are not common moments. Bad things happen to all of us. If I want to comfort myself with a bowl of ice-cream, that might be morally okay, but it shouldn't be confused with self-compassion. Self-compassion isn't about what you "deserve" or about entitlement. And self-compassion isn't the same thing as self-pity, a focus on your own problems and the tendency to forget that those around you experience problems too. Life is difficult for everyone. Remembering that we all share the human experience will not only increase your compassion for others, but will also help you be gentler with yourself.

Self-Compassion: Not Artificial.

You don't tell yourself things you know aren't true. You don't tell yourself you are good at something when you don't feel this is accurate.

A Self-Compassionate Mind Doesn't Feel Sorry For Itself and Doesn't Justify or Excuse Itself.

If you're late for an appointment, self-compassion will suggest that instead of saying "I'm such a jerk," or "I can't help it, I'm always late," you might say: "Okay I figured out what got in the way of getting to my appointment on time, and now I know how to fix it." You'll feel encouraged. You might have some regret, but no self-recrimination.

See, the thing is this: getting down on yourself is like putting a hole in your gas tank. It just leaves you with less get-up-and-go so that you can't make the changes you need to make.

It's entirely ineffective as a problem-solving method. And it's hard on relationships. Without self-compassion you end up using others to prop yourself up, and this can wear out friendships. In addition, self-criticism can become seductive. We may believe that it will help us avoid worse harm, or perhaps will keep us safe on the straight and narrow. But bringing up painful incidents over and over in our memory only makes problems worse. Then we become vulnerable to depression and end up essentially paralyzed, unable to change or let go of the past.

Many people believe that the ticket to achievement is to be hard on themselves: if they are tougher on themselves, they will be more likely to take action and make the needed changes. But that kind of self-talk actually increases anxiety and hopelessness as well as eroding motivation. It's like using a cattle prod — in the short run it will get the cattle moving— but it doesn't create lasting motivation. So instead of kicking yourself when you make a mistake, try instead to gently understand why you might have made that mistake. Accept your inherent mortality and humanity, and recognize that you are not alone. We all make mistakes. Sometimes even two or three! Per year!

Self-Compassion: Not Self-Esteem.

The "self-esteem" idea is about feeling good about oneself, often in a way that relies on recent achievements, self-confidence or superiority. Self-compassion promotes emotional resilience in a way that self-esteem cannot. It's doing what's in your own best interest, gently and without letting yourself off the hook. People with high levels of self-compassion tend to take more personal responsibility than people with high self-esteem, and they have a more stable sense of self-worth. Because kindness to self doesn't fluctuate based on external circumstances, people with self-compassion are better able to buffer themselves against life stressors, are less likely to get angry at others and are more able to tolerate opinions that differ from their own.

So what IS self-compassion?

Treat Yourself With Warmth, Respect and Empathy.

Treat yourself the way you might treat someone you really love. Imagine you disagree with a close friend or are disappointed by his or her behavior. You probably don't outright reject that friend just because you had a disagreement. The compassionate approach would be to respect your friend's differences, and continue to accept him or her with respect and empathy.

So it is with yourself. You might disappoint yourself sometimes – and if so, I give you a hearty welcome to the human race! – but there's no use in rejecting yourself and wallowing in shame. This kind of suffering just gets in the way of change.

Doing What is in Your Own Best Interest.

Please understand me in this point: self-compassion is not to be confused with selfish-ness. Self-compassion allows you to focus on living more effectively by doing what works. Often this means taking better care of your body, being kinder to those you love and generally being a nicer human being.

You are nicer to those around you when you can be nicer to yourself. The two ways of being are deeply connected, and not just because you are more stressed out and irritable with others when you've been harsh with yourself all week. When you can view yourself with more compassion, it's easier to view others with compassion as well. Rather than condemning yourself and those around you for their faults, you'll see the bigger picture. We are all of us wounded warriors, and there are understandable and compelling reasons for our foibles and failures. If you interpret another's behavior as an offense to you, or something designed to hurt you, it's likely you will also interpret your own behavior harshly, and vice versa. The reality is that most people don't act — they react. They react out of fear and out of a need to protect themselves.[fff]

Dr. Neff, self-compassion researcher at UT-Austin[ggg], proposes that self-compassion is made of three key components:

- **Self-kindness:** being warm and understanding about your own

---

[fff] For a very complete and life-changing insight on this problem, read the book "Bonds That Make Us Free", by C. Terry Warner.

[ggg] Dr. Neff also provides a number of helpful resources on her website, self-compassion.org. I recommend that my clients use the guided self-compassion meditation exercises found on that website.

---

difficulties and pain, rather than being harshly self-critical

- **Common humanity**: recognizing that, as humans, we all have imperfections and make mistakes. It's framing our frailties in terms of our shared humanity.

- **Mindfulness:** taking a non-judgmental stance toward any emotions you might have. Seeing things clearly without ignoring and without exaggerating.

Self-compassion isn't weakness. In fact, research demonstrates that people who are kind and gentle to themselves are better able to handle stress, and they recover more quickly from difficult life events. People with higher levels of self-compassion have a higher sense of self-efficacy and are less likely to fear failure. Even better, they tend to be more successful in achieving personal goals (such as quitting smoking). And of course, people with higher levels of self-compassion are much less likely to be depressed or anxious. A quote from Dr. Neff adds a further dimension: "Another advantage of self-compassion is that it is available precisely when self-esteem fails us – when we fall flat on our face, embarrass ourselves, or otherwise come in direct contact with the imperfection of life."

> *Self-indulgence is a counterfeit for happiness.*

How Self-Compassion Changes the Game

Self compassion is one of the latest "new" concepts in mental health that has been put forward as a therapy in and of itself. Self-compassion is a way of being kind to oneself without being self-indulgent. Self-compassion seeks what is in one's own best interests, not necessarily what one may actually be "in the mood for." It is learning to find an affection for the self and a level of consistent positive self-regard.

One primary path to developing better self-compassion is through self-mastery. Self-mastery (or self-discipline) is essentially the ability to get yourself to do what you have committed to do. It's the ability to follow through on goals, to be in control of your own appetites and how you use your time. It's the ability to get yourself to go to bed when you know you should, not when you decide you want to. It's the ability to get yourself to exercise or to say no to that french fry.

Most importantly, self-mastery is learned *in the context of self-compassion,* because otherwise it doesn't work in the long run. If you are interested in long-term change, you must develop self-mastery that grows out of self-respect, not out of guilt. Guilt will kill you when you use it as a motivator rather than as an in-the-moment guide to what you believe is right.[hhh]

Let me encourage you to develop a sense of competence or accomplishment. I might have a sense of mastery when I complete my taxes, weed a bed of lettuce, make the bed, or finish an

---

[hhh] It powerfully erodes motivation.

assignment. Without the ability to be in charge of our own appetites and desires, we have a hard time respecting ourselves. This lack of self-respect cannot be ignored and talked away through constantly pumping up of the self (e.g., "I'm okay even though I ate that half-gallon of ice cream.") Deep down, whenever we fail ourselves, we have that sense that we cannot rely on ourselves to follow through on our commitments, even our commitments to ourselves. Our self-respect grows as we learn to keep our commitments.

You may not have a well-grounded sense of self-respect, a sense that you are worthy of kept commitments. Act as if you do. The truth is that we already *are* full of worth as human beings, whether or not we gobble down a gallon—or even four—of ice cream per day. Our actions are independent of our worth, and there is nothing that we can do to lower (or increase) our infinite worth as human beings[iii].

In addition to a realization of worth, we need a sense of self-mastery in order to respect ourselves. To that end, it is crucial to learn how to get ourselves to be in charge of our appetites, desires and time. Only then can we learn to trust ourselves. This all must be done only in the context of self-compassion, and not, not, not! in the context of lashing out in self-hatred or cruelty or anger at the self.

Don't fall into the trap of believing that a life of self-discipline is a life without pleasure. A

[iii] Thanks, Mack, for sharing this wisdom with me many years ago. It changed my life.

disciplined, self-compassionate life can be full of joy and pleasure. On the other hand, self-indulgence is a counterfeit for happiness. Believing that you can find lasting happiness in satisfying your sweet tooth or indulging your urge to engage in activities that are not in your best interest is the kind of belief that will fall flat. Think about it. The solution is to learn to associate the feeling of pleasure with the things that are also in your best self-interest. Create a place in your brain where pleasure can be found in connection with healthful things, and you can thereby learn to "indulge" in exercise, vegetables and balanced sleep.

There is a great deal of science to support the idea that change happens best through positive reinforcement. Punishment may result in short-term compliance, but punishment also results in resentment and lack of motivation. Likewise, if we seek to change ourselves by whipping ourselves to do better out of shame, our coercive efforts will backfire in the long term. I have seen a number of folks who, after years of pushing themselves harshly, found themselves so completely out of motivation, so weary of their sense of failure, that they were nearly allergic to any expectations whatsoever. Indeed, they were deeply depressed. How could they have been otherwise?

> When we find ourselves worshipping "feel better" more than "do better," we also find that we have to artificially prop up our good feelings.

Self-mastery is not a popular treatment in the world of therapies designed to keep the patient comfortable and propped up in fantasies of "I'm okay, you're okay, we're all okay, no matter what." Self-mastery doesn't really mix well with pop psychotherapy's version of moral and behavioral relativism (i.e., you don't have to do anything, there are no requirements, except that you just feel better).

Let's not ignore the underlying truth that how you feel about yourself relates entirely to what you do. How you feel about yourself, however, is not related to your inherent worth.

Doing What's in Your Best Interest

To live self-compassionately you have to do what is in your best interest, not what will make you feel safe.

Yes, failure is safe. Failure is safe because it is predictable. Anything other than failure offers a possibility that cannot be predicted, and will therefore scare you into finding ways to fail. This is not in your best interest.

Don't Use Others as a Safety Dance

Remember the song, *Safety Dance?* You can dance the safety dance if you want to. It just isn't a happy dance.

Sometimes we deceive ourselves into thinking we can't hack life alone. We give up our willingness to do what is needed and buy into stories that absolve ourselves of personal responsibility. For example, you might rely on a medication to work for you so you feel happy. You might count on your therapist, your spouse, your children, or even your dog to make you feel better. Too many in our culture swallow the story that their depression or anxiety is out of their control and just dropped on them from the sky.[iii] This very passive approach almost always ends in greater unhappiness for the individual. It doesn't work in the long run.

Relationships (both with humans and pets) can create good feelings. However, a relationship cannot last if it is only a prop for your sense of well-being.

Developing self-mastery requires doing a number of hard things. First you have to learn to be completely honest with yourself. Honesty means factual accuracy – NOT harshness. Honesty means seeing the reality of the current situation.

There's a great analogy in the book *Five Things We Cannot Change* (by David Richo) that I love to share with my patients. I'll paraphrase it: Seeing reality for *what it really is,* is like deciding to turn around in the saddle and face the direction your horse is already going.

Dude, you are IN reality. Whether or not you choose to SEE reality is up to you.

When you distort reality in ways that make you feel safe, what you are doing is essentially ascribing blame elsewhere for your problems. Blaming requires victimhood and victimhood keeps you stagnant.

Lots of people have gone through terrible things in life that shouldn't have happened. You may be one of them. It's very likely that whatever happened to you wasn't something you could

---

[iii] The "chemical imbalance" hypothesis has been so thoroughly disproved elsewhere that I will not address it here.

You Can Let Other People Make Your Life Difficult

You have a choice in how you interact with difficult people:

1. You can WILL them to change. You can spend tons of time thinking about how they should or shouldn't be the way that they are. You can try to fix them. This is miserable.

2. You can simply give up and let them be the way they are. You can move away. You can distance yourself. This way you aren't around the person. This is slightly less miserable.

3. You can have a superficial relationship with the person. This is still a form of distancing. Still miserable.

4. You can be with the other person in a way that invites change through your willingness to show up as who you really are, complete with your feelings, your caring and your unprotected heart. This is hard. This doesn't fix the person. But it inspires a different relationship with the person.

---

have controlled at the time. But staying stuck in that place only keeps you miserable, so let go of the blaming. Know that letting go of blame is not the same thing as approving the bad things that happened to you. Trust that you can take charge of your life now. To do so requires seeing reality clearly, gathering courage and taking responsibility, but it's the only way toward finding happiness.

What did you have for breakfast yesterday? Remember? You can choose to re-experience that same breakfast over and over in your mind. It can gain a lot of power over you if you do. You can become a victim to how that breakfast ruined your lunch. Or you can let it go and find a new life to focus on. Whatever happened to you can either stay in your focus or be let go of through mental self-discipline – learning to be in charge of what you are paying attention to in your mind. Mindfulness practice is how you learn to take charge of your focus. Seeing reality as it really is creates responsibility. Then you decide to take charge of the outcomes in your life, and you see that you actually can change the behaviors that create those outcomes.

An Example: What I Think I Do and What I'm Actually Doing

Here's an example. I might feel that I am doing a great job of taking care of my health. I think that I eat mostly good food, I don't ever eat fast food, I eat hardly any processed food, and I try to get to the gym multiple times per week. But I am still plagued by problems. My blood sugar is out of control. My weight is far too high. I'm tired. I'm irritable. I have trouble sleeping. Coming to reality means that I take a look at what I am *actually* doing instead of my perception of how well I'm doing. For instance, if you took a look at how many times my gym ID was actually swiped at the gym in the past four months, you would find that number to be 3 times total, and not 48. If you look at what I actually ate this week, you'd find that in addition to a number of vegetables and fruits, I've also downed a quart of Ben & Jerry's (and I'm allergic to dairy), multiple chocolate bars, a chocolate croissant and an apple-cider donut. Instead of drinking at least three quarters of a gallon of water per day, I've been lucky to down 48 ounces and on some days it's been less than that. I think of myself as getting to bed each night at 10 pm, but that is just my ideal. If I had been wearing an actigraph (a device that measures sleep) the data would show that I'm falling asleep on average around midnight, waking up for an hour or two in the middle of the night and dragging myself out of bed far later than my ideal of 6:40 a.m. So my actual sleep, exercise and diet do not match up to my fantasy of what I'd like to think I'm doing.

Doesn't it make sense, then, that my body isn't fooled!

Of course I'm still struggling with the symptoms of poor sleep, lack of exercise, weight, irritability, high blood sugar, etc. Those symptoms are not coming out of the blue. They are happening because my "good behaviors" are only intentions, not reality. At least, not a consistent reality.

Learning how to make intentions a consistent reality is part of developing self-mastery. And learning to have self-mastery works only in the context of self-compassion. You learn to do these things AS A KINDNESS to yourself, and NOT AS A "SHOULD."

This is a sign that I've made for clients and put next to my own notes for self-improvement: "Do it as a kindness, not as a 'should.'" When I go to the gym out of kindness for myself, my entire sense of willingness and choice is deeply affected. If I made myself go to the gym through using shame or some other form of coercion, I might be relieved afterward that I exercised but I won't find a resilient sense of motivation growing out of that experience. I'll just be able to get to short-term compliance. I may exercise to avoid self recrimination, but this way doesn't result in self-discipline. Instead, it's a reliable way to erode my motivation.

Remember the principle that people who exercise for life are people who enjoy the exercise? This is why: The exercise they are doing doesn't feel like a punishment!

Okay, so the first thing is to see reality. Next you want to change your actual behaviors to match up better with what you know is in your best interest. Here, it's important to avoid "shoulds." As the famous Albert Ellis says, "Stop shoulding all over yourself!"

The "shoulds" are coercive and erode motivation. You want to protect your precious motivation resource and nurture it into something resilient. So stop "shoulding" on yourself (and others). Let go and become far more free and able to change behavior out of choice and not shame. Track your use of the very word "should" and see what I mean.

> *Let go of the idea that it's not fair. It doesn't matter. It's not like the Fair Fairy is going to eventually hear you and magically change your life.*

You'll also want to get rid of those feelings of "it's not fair!" Sure, it's not fair that you may have to work harder than the others to get the same results. It's not fair that you have to give up more to get the same results. The longer you stay stuck in how not fair it is, the longer you stay stuck in not getting results. So give it up. Let go of the idea that it's not fair. It doesn't matter. It's not like the Fair Fairy is going to eventually hear you and magically change your life.

When you let go of the "it's not fair" or the "it shouldn't be this way," then you can experience the feelings underneath your discouragement. You'll be swimming through some sadness and pain, but the sadness and pain is manageable when you let go of how unfair it feels. Just experience the sadness and pain cleanly. You can't drown in it unless you really try hard. The water is only 3 feet high. It's as if there's a pool you have to wade through to get to the other side – the side where you can be over the sadness and pain. Every time you start thinking about how unfair it all is you get stuck at the entrance to the pool, again and again.

Start small. Nurture your desire. Cheerlead yourself. Offer yourself kind encouragement even if it feels uncomfortable at first. These changes are made in the context of kindness, affection and encouragement.

Self-compassion doesn't just drop on you out of the sky. It's a behavior that anyone can learn. Really. It's just a matter of practice. Even if you are beginning with very little self-compassion, if you practice this behavior correctly, and often enough, you will develop the skill of self-compassion. I guarantee it!

And your life will, indeed, get better.

Chapter Fifteen

Act Yourself Into Change

We try to talk ourselves into changing. We use all kinds of talk. We yell, we wheedle, we moan and groan. It doesn't work. What works is when we <u>act</u> ourselves into change, behave ourselves into change. What works is developing one small habit at a time until we are good and changed. The ability to change is created through practicing.

When we try over and over to simply talk ourselves into change, we get discouraged because it doesn't work. In order to protect our tender feelings, we then have to come up with explanations about why we didn't end up actually changing. We either blame ourselves or blame someone or something else for why we did not create change. When we blame ourselves, we may attack our worth, our personality, or our motivation. We may say we are lazy or undisciplined. We feel helpless. We get discouraged: "What's wrong with me! I can't do it!"

Worse, we may start to believe we are not capable of change. This explanation entirely lets us off the hook because if we aren't capable of change then we don't need to invest any work in changing. We protect our fragile egos by either blaming ourselves (we can't help it because we can't change) or blaming others (we can't help it because we have no power). Both of these approaches create and increase helplessness, and decrease our ability to take responsibility for our lives. Now, please understand that I'm not suggesting that you should be able to regenerate your limbs through the force of your cheerful will! I'm saying that, no matter your circumstances, you can still take responsibility for creating health-promoting, happiness-promoting change.

It's a mind-body thing. In order to have a chance at change, you have to approach it from the perspective of seeing yourself as a whole healthy person standing firmly on that three-legged stool. In case you need me to beat a dead horse, this means it won't work to try to create change while simultaneously ignoring sleep, eating and exercise.

Here's more irony – when we are beating ourselves up about not changing (we might say either I'm bad or it's Life's fault and both of these

> *We try to talk ourselves into change when what we need to do is behave ourselves into change.*

methods of being a victim are problematic), we are nonetheless engaged in change — it's just change that is counter-productive. All our talk without action results in decreased self-efficacy and sometimes self-hate. Self-efficacy is a sense of capability, a confidence that one can do what one sets out to do. Decreasing our self-efficacy was not our original intent, but when we attack our efficacy through harsh self-talk, we decrease our power to be different than we are, and increase our misery.

Stop it!

Small Habits Create Change

You probably know some people who can create change. You may think of them as remarkably self-disciplined, or just naturally better than the rest of us. It's as if their self-discipline qualities fell from the sky, and the rest of us are just not as favored or as good. We think, "Oh wow! I could never count on myself to do that." Because we think of these effective people as belonging to a different class of humans, we don't let ourselves see the truth: they are simply more effective than we are because of their behaviors.

Simply establishing a habit — one small little thing — is the handy wedge you need to get that door open to the New You. It's all about action, baby.

But something gets in the way. What gets in the way of that life-enhancing action is usually your thoughts.

How many times have you wanted to be different? How many times have you studied about the changes you want to make? If I got the body that came from wanting, I'd be a pretty hot mama. And if I got the body based on what I know, I'd be unbelievable. But change doesn't result from wanting, learning or thinking. Change only comes about from doing.

It's Not About Wanting, Learning or Thinking, It's About Choosing, and then, Doing

Many of my clients aren't used to having to actually do the work of change. I tell them that this is because they are too smart for their own good! Since they never had to work hard in school in order to achieve good results, they never learned that working hard is connected to getting results. Instead, they learned to coast. They created achievements without really working for them. Then, when coasting stopped working for them later in life, they got frustrated and discouraged. They often blamed themselves or blamed others rather than identifying the underlying problem. You see, the only tool for change that they ever got any practice with in their formative years was the "figure-it-out-you're-smart" tool. Whereas this may be a great tool for understanding calculus, it's not so effective when applied to other, non-academic life areas. Thus, when "figuring it out" only leads to a brick wall, these people are reluctant to let go of their "figure-it-out-tool." Instead, they beat their heads on that brick wall.

The frequent result is depression and strained relationships.

Our Stories About Life Keep Us Stagnant

Here's another example of how we avoid actual behaviors in our attempts to change. This is my story —well, one of them anyway! It served to protect my poor fragile ego from the real consequences of the behaviors I wanted to remain blind to. The story I told myself kept me from action. It has kept me from making needed changes in my life. Bear in mind, for most of my life I was largely unconscious of how this underlying story affected me. It was hard for me to read it in myself until I got the help to see it.[kkk] The story was this:

> I am fated to keep failing! God has (kindly) arranged this for me in order to protect me from the evils of success. Since all successful people are secretly jerks, it's much safer to stay a failure because that way I don't risk being a real jerk[lll].

When I (unconsciously) failed in order to (unconsciously) protect myself from becoming a successful jerk, I was able to have the fantasy that I wasn't really "failing." The only thing about my "story" that I was consciously aware of was

---

[kkk] I want to thank Peter Lotterhos and Transformational Mind Dynamics for helping me identify my stories.

[lll] Chilling, isn't it? And guess what...I can still be a jerk, whether or not I am a failure or a success!!

the fleeting thought, "It probably won't work because that's how things turn out for me." But the reality that I was blind to seeing was this: I was being a fail martyr for the cause of non-jerks everywhere who don't succeed in order to stay humble. What a crock!

Since I didn't trust myself to be able to stay grounded in the face of success, when success would nonetheless happen I would feel either as though I didn't deserve it, or I couldn't connect my successes with my real self. I would not allow a conscious connection between my actions and any real changes that resulted. Consequently I often felt like a fraud. I had little confidence that I could actually finish what I started.

My story is an old story, a common story. I learned it while young from my parents, and I'm 100% certain that they did not intend to teach it to me! But because I learned it young, it ran deep in my heart and my mind. You have stories that you learned too, from parents who probably did not intend to teach them. Until you find out what they are, they will continue to affect your ability to make the changes you want in your life.

Do you see how this fantasy about being fated to fail made it easier for me to not give 100% to my exercise efforts? If I believed it wouldn't work anyway because success was not there for me, why try harder? And why open my eyes to the painful truth that my exercise efforts were, in reality, less than 100%.

Failure Fate, Meet the Good Girl!

Increased self-awareness in the process of ferreting out the lies in my self-deceptive thinking took my insights to the next level. I discovered that, in addition to thinking I had Failure Fate, I also had a Must Be a Good Girl disease.

Yowza.

The only way to be a failure *and* be a good girl was to have awesome excuses. And I had truly awesome excuses: My feet hurt. I had Lyme disease. I didn't want to hurt her feelings. Et cetera. When I was little, I used to tell my friends to call me if they needed an excuse and I'd come up with a doozy!

Honestly, my excuse-making behavior was very helpful when I was little. It represented my little brain doing its best to survive in my world. We all have these kinds of survival-oriented learned behavioral patterns, based on our past. The problem is that no matter how helpful these kinds of behaviors might have been when we were all seven years old, they stop being helpful when we're grown up.

In the end game, all the excuses in the world — no matter how legitimate — don't change the eventual outcomes. It's not like the Excuse Fairy says, "Oh, I see. You were only doing what you had to do. So I'll save you from the consequences resulting from your choices!"

Here's an example. For years I'd wanted to lose weight and become more physically fit. I'd tried many things and hadn't yet gotten the results I wanted. Whenever I engaged in pro-fitness behavior, I would run into challenges. Everyone does. But instead of working through those challenges, I would come up with excuses about why it was okay to fail[mmm]. But I wasn't failing because was okay to fail! I was failing because I was using excuses to get out of behavior that's just hard to do. And I was not even aware that this was the reality of my life. I was attached to my belief that the reason I wasn't at the gym was that my feet hurt too much. This attachment to beliefs about why we do what we do is a very human thing to have, and it really gets in the way of our achieving our dreams.

There was another style of excuse that popped up for me. If you classify the previous excuses described above as in the style of "I can't," then these further excuses would be categorized as in the style of "I haven't had this experience yet, and I deserve it," or "I might never get this again in my whole life!" This second style of excuses arose from my having felt deprived in the past. They were my mind's attempts to keep me safe from being deprived again, but my mind was fooling me about what deprivation was and what the actual danger of it might be *now*, in this very present moment. "Note to brain: the lack of that cookie[nnn] is *not* going to result in death!"

Deprivation and Change

When you approach change from a culture of deprivation, it's actually neurologically harder to make good choices. You see, in a culture of

---

[mmm] It really *is* okay to fail as long as you are aware of it. Failing means you are engaging in action. The more you fail, the higher your success rate becomes.

[nnn] The basil-pepper chocolate truffle, on the other hand... Visit Laughing Moon Chocolates to feel my pain.

abundance, when the brain is faced with many choices, it's much easier to make choices that are in line with your end goals. But when the brain is faced with very few choices, it becomes harder to choose well. It's actually neurologically more difficult, not just more difficult because of your past or because you are hungry in the present moment.

Being raised in a culture of deprivation causes the brain to become literally less efficient. In its attempt to protect you, your brain learns to shout "GET IT WHILE YOU CAN!" and it's hard to hear that there just might be another, better choice. It doesn't occur to you that you could think, "I don't actually need it so I don't *want* to get it at all." But just because it's harder to hear that freeing choice doesn't mean the Excuse Fairy will "bippity-boppity-boo" you a different, unrelated consequence.

When you play Monopoly, in order to get out of jail you have to pay the price. There is no other way.

Likewise, the consequences of your past behaviors are what exist in your life right now! If you don't like those consequences, blame or excuses won't change them for you, even if blame and excuses make you feel better in the short run. The only things that will change those consequences are your future actions.

Our Superpower Ability to Be Unaware Is Not So Super

Humans have superpower abilities to be unaware of their unconscious thinking and unaware of how their behavior follows those lines of unconscious, unexamined thoughts. It's a perfect storm. Your perfect storm might look a little different from mine, but the result remains the same: *your unconscious thinking will consistently derail you from ever really following through on what's in your best interest.*

Don't get discouraged. Your brain can change. Behavior changes the brain very powerfully, and change can become easier for you through practice!

And the truth is that discouragement is something that you can choose either to nurture or to get rid of. If you are willing to work hard enough to attain some mental discipline (which I define as control over what thoughts you hang on to), you can learn to let go of discouragement. You can choose what you think about in any given moment. Random thoughts may pop up and knock on the door, asking to be entertained, but you are the one who answers the door. You are the one who decides which thoughts to invite in for dinner. The more you practice mindfulness,°°° the more you are able to be in charge of your thoughts.

And that's critical to creating the life changes that will be in your best self-interest.

Here's an example: My family is eating homemade burgers, seasoned with a little Herbes de Provence, and layered with some bacon ketchup, smoked onion mustard and fresh heirloom tomatoes. I'm choosing to stick to a 100% vegan diet for the day. I plan to eat a

---

°°° See every book Jon Kabat-Zinn has ever written.

Portobello mushroom. Wow, I am so good! Wow, I am so deprived! I start feeling sorry for myself as I prepare their food as well as mine. My taste buds are screaming for hamburgers because the fact is I dearly love hamburgers, and I've never yet tried bacon ketchup or smoked onion mustard! But wait! I stop the "want" thoughts. To begin with, I ignore my taste buds. <u>I also command my thoughts to ignore them too.</u> In fact, I don't allow myself to think thoughts like "Ooh, that would taste so good," etc. End result: the thought "I wish I could eat that hamburger" indeed knocked at the door, but I didn't answer.

This is the key: – I am changing by disciplining my thinking. I don't allow myself to wallow in the fantasy of how that hamburger would taste. My thoughts stay focused on broiling my Portobello mushroom with some red onions and creating a fantastically tasty tahini-garlic sauce.ppp When I taste it, it is awesome. I mean it really blows me away. I love it.

Since I gave myself permission (mentally and physically) to enjoy the alternative, and I did not focus on what I was missing, I was able to actually taste and thoroughly enjoy what was there on my plate.

Our Brains Lie to Us

When we think about change, we often worry that there will never be any pleasure again in our lives. Ever.

In this, our brains lie to us. They tell us that the only pleasures available are those we've

---

ppp Thank you, *Eat to Live*, by Joel Furhman. Great recipes.

Taste Buds Change!

I have some friends who make their daughter try foods she doesn't like every time they serve them. It could well be every week! They say "You never know. Your taste buds can change, so you have to see if you like it yet."

They are so right! Research tells us that indeed our taste preferences really do change over time. The tastes we enjoy at age 7 will not be the same tastes we have at age 37. We can become more "sophisticated" tasters if we only keep trying new foods. It's when we get stuck on the brain lie that "you don't like mushrooms, ever" that you refuse to try them.

Moms typically give up after their children refuse a particular food a few times. But we know that it can take about 10 tastes of a new food (different occasions) before taste buds can accommodate the new food, especially if "palatability" of the food is low (hint: sugar and fat have high palatability). Think about a mom's typical attitude to serving cabbage vs. ice cream. The child has to overcome palatability aspects AND mom's attitude. Taste buds are just taste buds. Your brain creates flavor. So modeling enjoyment of healthy foods really helps.

P.S. You have taste buds on the roof of your mouth, in your stomach and in your throat. And the life cycle of a taste bud is only about 2 weeks. Interesting, eh?

already experienced. Surely nothing else, besides what we've had in the past, could be very pleasurable — like Portobello mushroom sandwiches[qqq], for instance. In my case, I'd had them before, and I'd experienced how good they

[qqq] Or like success, right?

were, but my brain still wouldn't believe! It was looking at a past in which hamburgers were enjoyed more frequently than Portobello sandwiches, simply because I didn't eat many Portobello sandwiches during the first forty years of my life!

You can't always trust the "want" part of your brain. The "want" part doesn't use logic, doesn't predict outcomes with foresight and has no clue what's in your best interest. The want part simply wants. It lives in the now, and doesn't have any conception of the future. It is able to completely overwhelm the logical thinking parts of your brain with incessant wanting, just as the blare of a smoke alarm preferentially gets your attention over the quiet words of your spouse. For example, it may tell you to eat things that will make you feel rotten. It may tell you to smoke and ignore impending cancer. It would not recognize the concept of "your best interest" if you wrote it in bright red neon!

Your Diet Affects Your Concept of "Your Best Interest"

One of my favorite research studies illustrates this point.[190] Scientists divided rats into three groups. One group ate regular rat food. The other two groups had access to a "cafeteria" diet that was a buffet of sugary, chocolately yumminess. Cheesecake, chocolate, pudding, pound cake, bacon and sausage were all parts of this buffet. One of the two groups of buffet rats had access to the cafeteria for an hour per day. The other group had access for up to 23 hours per day. The researchers then measured how much reward it took to get the three groups of rats to keep running on a treadmill. One of the results of the study was that the rats with 23-hour per day access to the pig-out cafeteria required significantly more rewards to do the same tasks that the other rats did for more normal rewards. Apparently the high-fat, high-sugar diet disrupted the pig-out rats' brain reward circuits enough that what used to be rewarding for them was no longer so rewarding.

Scientists next examined whether the rats' knowing that certain negative outcomes were imminent would result in any eating behavior changes. The researchers taught all the rats to associate a certain light with a mild electric shock. All the rats learned that when they saw this light, a shock was about to happen. Once the rats learned this, the researchers let all three groups of rats into the cafeteria area. It was a yummy-fest for every rat in the study and they all began to chow down. After a bit, the researchers showed the light signaling imminent shock. Two-thirds of the rats ran away. The other third stayed and kept eating, despite knowing they'd be shocked any second! The group that was willing to put up with electric shock in order to keep eating cheesecake was the group of rats that previously had been allowed nearly unlimited access to the fat and sugar-fest.

When people become obese, the body undergoes many changes. One of these changes is that it becomes harder to regulate fat intake. What this means is that obese people eat more fat than their bodies need to eat. New research shows that the mouth and gut are less able to sense fatty acids when individuals become obese.

One of the things that helps the body feel full is its ability to sense fat in food. This helps tell the brain to stop eating. So if becoming obese also impairs "fatty acid chemoreception" (fancy words for the brain's ability to sense when you've eaten enough fat), your brain won't give you as clear a message to stop eating as your thinner companions get from their less impaired brains.

When your brain is stuck in Want, it doesn't do a good job of identifying what's in your best interest. And when your brain has been smacked with a high fat, high sugar food fest, it's much harder to get yourself to find pleasure in other things. Not only that, but motivation to change and self-awareness of thinking and behavior both become much more elusive.

Getting Out of Stuck-ness: Look "Out Loud"

One of the most effective ways my past self kept me from being aware of my rationalizing was that I was too afraid to really look at my belief that God was creating failure as a kindness to me. It was as though I couldn't question that belief, because questioning that would be like questioning God. My brain totally faked me out on that one! So it was a major breakthrough for me to understand that this belief was just a belief and actually had NOTHING to do with God at all. Finally realizing this was a big deal. It set me free of that unfounded thought. I began to recognize it as simply a story my brain had come up with to make it easier for me so I could keep doing what I was doing and still be a Good Girl. How did I free myself of the power those unrecognized beliefs were holding over me? I had to look at them *Out Loud.*

Just thinking about it didn't do the job. I had to write it out, say it out loud, discuss it, admit it, and "own" it. Of course I found myself wanting to minimize my faulty thinking. It's downright embarrassing to be "Out Loud" about any of these kinds of beliefs at first, because most of us think we'll be rejected for being "so stupid." But the fear of embarrassment was just another obstacle that was getting in my way.

My kind husband listened to me as I started practicing looking Out Loud. His response — "Wow. That's really messed up."

Right?!! It helps to hear the truth. What a relief!

Through repetitive practice, I became better at doing the behaviors necessary to create the changes I wanted in my life. And even though I would often get sucked back unawares into my same old story, every time I Looked Out Loud I gained more practice in getting out of the lies. I got faster at detecting my faulty thinking in a way that created power –- the power to choose to change.

Resolve now to start the stopping of the behavior of bemoaning your lack of change. Bemoaning doesn't work, it's not very entertaining for yourself and it's not at all entertaining for others! It simply results in more discouragement.

But I Can't! I Have No Discipline!

We are remarkably self-disciplined when it comes to wearing clothing. We wear clothing all the time while we do errands, or are otherwise out of the house. Nobody gets to work and says, "Gosh, I got up late and I just didn't have time to get dressed. At all. So I'm buck naked here. Boy, this will be a little awkward when the boss walks in!" No, we all have a habit of putting some sort of clothing on before going to work. See my point? It's a habit. We have it. We made it. It's pretty dang reliable. Said another way, we have excellent self-discipline in that area. We really are in control.

But if you look at the things we aren't doing that are in our best interest, we somehow want to believe we are not in control.

What I'm saying is this: change is possible! Saying you can take responsibility is altogether different from saying that you should be ashamed! Realizing you can do something different in order to get a different outcome is not at all the same thing as shaming yourself by thinking that you must have intended to have this negative outcome all along.

You probably didn't wake up saying "Gosh, I want to be fat!" I certainly know I didn't. But my undisciplined behaviors didn't match my intention to not be fat. Our behaviors are the very things that keep any of us in poor physical shape.

So being overweight isn't a curse. It's a result. It's simply the outcome of your behaviors. Perhaps you have tried over and over to lose weight and it hasn't worked. My guess is that this outcome is because what you are doing is simply not effective. So instead of bemoaning your lack of change, let's look at changing what you are doing. Make the effort to track what you are actually doing. Analyze what you're doing to see if your behaviors are getting you the outcomes you want. Don't make this process about feeling bad or shameful. Do that and you have entirely missed the point. In addition, you become very vulnerable to emotionally eating your way out of your misery and consequently staying overweight. What naturally follows is your crafting a rationalizing explanation about your body that bears some similarity (in function, if not in content) to my story about Failure Fate earlier in the chapter.

Sure, new behaviors generally set off anxiety. You can decide to just be anxious and do the behaviors anyway. It's kind of like saying "Damn the torpedoes! Full steam ahead!"

Mind-Body Connections That Trip Us Up

When your body is out of shape, your mind is out of shape too. For example, let's say you set a goal to lose weight. I'm not talking about being movie-star thin when that's not a healthy shape for you. I'm talking about losing the weight that is over *your* healthy weight.

So let's say you choose to stop overeating as one method to lose weight. But the effects of obesity in your body get in the way of your good intentions. Obesity causes your gut to be less active in digestion, and causes your cephalic response to be impaired.

Cephalic response? What's that, you say?

A cephalic response occurs when your body reacts to sweet things *as if* they were calorically dense even if they contain zero calories. Your tongue senses sweetness and in turn, your pancreas quits making protein from your body reserves, and starts pumping out insulin so it can store the incoming excess blood sugar as fat. This insulin will not only make you hungrier (especially if you are actually eating zero calories) but will also increase fat storage. So even if you are drinking a zero calorie sweet drink, you will still gain weight. This process can happen in the body whether or not you are obese, but being obese makes it more likely.[191]

If you want to say that learning about this physiological mechanism means it's not your fault that you overeat, you can say that. It's just not helpful. What's more helpful is to recognize that the outcome of previous behavior has created a situation where it is harder to regulate food intake. You have to try extra hard to change your habits. You can choose to entirely quit

> One of the neurotransmitters involved in regulating hunger is serotonin. You may recognize that neurotransmitter from its most publicized role in depression. Doing things that boost serotonin levels will help you regulate food intake.
>
> Incidentally, do you know what else boosts serotonin levels? Willpower. Using willpower and increasing willpower through practice also increases serotonin.

eating all artificial sweeteners and drinking any sodas. This behavior will really help.

Here's the bottom line: You either do the behavior or you don't do it. Your factual behavior is the key to your being overweight and out of shape. Any other talk about it is simply talk that allows you to refuse to take responsibility, excuses your actions or keeps you stuck in the misery of being out-of-shape.

Oh no, you say. This is so very politically incorrect!

True. It's more politically correct to preach the word of Fat is Okay[rrr].

But when you wake up fat in the morning, your body isn't okay. You have poor energy. You get sick more frequently. You have more knee pain, higher levels of inflammation and your hormones are funky.

Your body doesn't lie. Your brain will lie to you all day, but your body doesn't lie.

Oh, wait. You think this method won't work for you. You think you are special and the things that work for other people don't work for you.

I hear you. I hear you hard.

As I became more aware of how I sabotaged my efforts to act in 100% alignment with my goals, I started to understand in a more powerful way how good I had been at fooling myself. I once was the queen of "that won't work for me." And the end result was what I'd had in front of me all along: a body that was out of shape.

[rrr] Again, I'm talking about weight that is over a healthy weight for YOU, not a socially determined ideal.

So I finally got wise to it. I changed my behaviors. Guess what? There was no "guarantee fail" in this game after all. Failure was all in my head.

Chapter Sixteen

Your Game Plan

No, no, no. Do not read this chapter first. It won't help you nearly as much. You are cheating yourself.

Thanks.

Imagine you hear me say, "Gosh, I hope I exercise today. I hope I sleep well tonight. I hope I eat healthy. I'm totally crossing my fingers. I'm really going to try."

What do you think? What are my chances?

Hoping and trying aren't doing. Neither will help me unless I start moving. So I'm going to blow my own mind and choose to actually *do* those things.

Today I am eating healthy, and going on a 30-minute walk, after which I'll do a 30-lap swim. Later I'll go to bed at 10:30 pm. I know what to do in order to make those things happen because I've practiced it. I'm not planning on it — I'm in the middle of doing it.

Now, I bet you believe me. I sound different because I'm not just hoping or trying. I'm doing.

But I Can't!

If you are stuck saying "I can't," part of the solution is to change your language. Eliminate that very word, "can't," for one. Say things like "I don't skip exercising." People who say "I don't ___ " tend to follow through on their commitments more frequently than people who say things like "I can't skip exercise."

"I can't" are words that limit you in every way. They even feel blah to say.

Try this. Say out loud "I want to eat healthy today."

Now try saying: "I choose to eat healthy today."

Feels better, doesn't it? In both cases (choose and don't vs. want and can't) you are telling your brain that you are in charge.

I remember years ago, when my kids were very small (one was a baby and the other was about 18 months old) I had this thought: "I can't go to choir practice. I have these two small babies and my husband is at work. So I can't do it." One day I stopped that thought and took a hard look at it. I realized that I was the only one saying I couldn't do it. No one else was telling me that. Instead of giving up before I started, I decided to try to find a solution. I chose to go anyway. I figured I'd hold the three month-old in my arms and sing while looking at someone else's music. The toddler could run around until she clearly needed to go home. I experimented to see how long I could last at choir practice. Sure, there were days where I was only there for 15 minutes. But I was able to do much more than I had thought I could. After a while I decided to stop going to choir practice. It wasn't because I couldn't do it. It was because I chose not to go. Big difference.

Connecting to Change

I like to identify three levels of change: intellectual, emotional and physical/behavioral. When you are in the intellectual level of change, you know what you need to do. You understand how to change. When you are in the emotional level of change, you know you really need to do it! You get in touch with the feeling that change must happen. When you are in the physical/behavioral level of change, you simply do it!

What level of change creates results? Behavioral change. Anything else is just glucose going around in the brain.

Don't be upset at yourself for being in a level that doesn't create real change. Be patient and self-compassionate. This means that you have become aware of where you are, you notice it and then you take steps to move on. It doesn't mean that you stay there and tell yourself it's okay to wallow (again, that's not self-compassion). You allow yourself to make mistakes in the context of actually doing, all the while continuing to like yourself. Making mistakes is crucial if you are interested in making any progress. So

> *When you are in the intellectual level of change, you know what you need to do. When you are in the emotional level of change, you really know you need to do it! When you are in the physical/behavioral level of change, you do it!*

when you fail, you notice what went wrong and then you fix it.

Besides, change is a process. You have to start in either the intellectual or emotional level before you are able to move onward to the behavioral level of change. Keep moving through the process rather than becoming stagnant. The longer you stay in the intellectual or emotional stages of change, the more you feel impotent about your ability to eventually change.

There's a Chinese proverb that states this telling truth: "If you want to know your past, look into your present conditions. If you want to know your future, look into your present actions."

If you don't ask yourself for real change, real change won't happen. If you are too afraid to make a difference, you won't make a difference. If I wrote this chapter wanting you to like me, I might pretend that health and lasting change really weren't hard to do! I might propose four easy steps, or a magic pill. But this won't work for you — you wouldn't get the results that you wanted in the long run, and you'd end up even more discouraged. My false popularity would disappear because it had been based on telling you what you wanted to hear so you could stay safe, not based on telling you what really works. What really works are actions that are often hard and anxiety-provoking!

I read in a recent magazine that people can sleep more with one simple change: just dim the lights 15 minutes before bedtime to stimulate melatonin. Or they could eat better by simply snacking every few hours to avoid hunger.

Easy, huh? What I'm saying here is that magic bullets like these are not enough. Sure, these suggestions aren't hard to implement, but chances are you need interventions with more power if the goal you are reaching for is to actually make a difference in your life.

Look at it this way: If you eat 9 bags of corn chips per week instead of 10, you are eating healthier. But is that going to create the difference you want?

I doubt it.

It's not popular to assert that real change requires that you engage in hard work by giving up the things that are keeping you stuck. We Americans are big fans of both having and eating the proverbial cake. So I'm not going to comfort you with the idea that you can keep all the cookies, do a few stomach crunches and in 10 years there will be a magic pill that will do all the work for you.

> *You only need to change as much as it takes in order to get the outcomes you want.*

No. You only need to change as much as it takes to get the outcomes you want. For me, 15 minutes of dimmed lights before bed just ain't gonna cut it. Ever.

The Goal is Results, Not Rules

When you set up your change strategy so that it's about sticking to set rules, it's hard to individualize it so it will work for you. For example, if I want to get up to running a 5K and I set a goal to run a certain amount each day, when obstacles arise it will be harder for me to make needed adjustments. When I learn that I am responsible for the results, and not for merely sticking to my rules, I will plan and execute more effectively. I can make needed adjustments that will keep me focused on moving toward my goal rather than confining myself to being a good or bad girl.

Here are some tips you can use as you design your own program.

Thoughts on Change

1. Don't change too much at once

You want changes that last, not a frenzy that kills you. So start small. Pick one thing and divide it into four steps. Then do just the first step. Practice that step until it becomes easy, then add the second step. Continue until you have added all the steps to complete your behavior. Along the way remind yourself that you are doing this as a kindness to yourself, not a "should". Notice how good you feel about the change you are making. Notice anything that is positive.

If it turns out you're not meeting your goals, evaluate the situation and adapt your plan. For example, if I want to feel like my house is cleaner each day, I might start by simply making my bed. If I can't manage to make my bed, I'll need to assess why that is — and likely it's because I am far too fatigued to function very well in any area. If that's the case, I need to work on the fatigue instead of beating myself up with "I can't even make my own stupid bed." If I can't manage to make my own bed, there's a darn good reason for it. Identifying that reason is more effective than getting down on myself and further destroying my motivation.

2. Use Pleasure and Rewards to Your Benefit

Part of being a grown-up is learning (and by this I mean teaching yourself) to enjoy the things that are in your best interest. Instead of letting your pleasure rest in those things that are merely self-indulgent, practice loving the things that are actually good for you.

I have a friend who loves to go to sleep at night. I don't love it. I prefer to stay awake, bleary-eyed and doing whatever I can to avoid falling asleep. But I listened to what she was saying and took it to heart. I practiced enjoying going to bed. I pretended that I was my friend. It really helped. I could see her point. I found out that going to bed can be full of pleasure.

Don't hesitate to use rewards simply because you think you are too grown up to need them. You don't have to give yourself a cookie, for goodness sake! A reward is simply anything that will

---

Rewards to Consider:

• *Telling yourself "Great job!"*

• *Getting another person to tell you "Great job!"*

• *Music (downloading a song, etc.)*

• *A freshly sliced tomato with sea salt*

• *Playing a card game with friends*

• *Making a strawberry lemonade (stevia, 1 lemon, 2 strawberries, 2 cups of water and a powerful blender).*

• *A dollar in a special account for you to buy something you've wanted.*

• *Standing in the sun and relaxing.*

• *A phone call to a friend.*

increase the likelihood that you will repeat that behavior again.

On the other hand, especially when you are at the beginning of a behavior change and just starting to nurture a brand new behavior pattern, there will be some occasions when you don't want to do the new behavior despite having a reward waiting for you. You may decide that rewards don't actually work. You may be tempted to give up.

> *Giving up merely guarantees that results won't come. Ever.*

Sometimes you do need better rewards. But most of the time what I think happens is that people think themselves out of behaviors. Rewards truly help the simple "want" part of the brain learn that Behavior "X" leads to Outcome "Y." But the complicated part of your brain can easily get in the way of that process. Just do the behavior. Don't beat yourself with a stick. Don't tell yourself you better do it, or else! Don't even tell yourself that if you do it you can have a reward. That won't work very well for the tough times, because there will always be some days where no reward feels good enough to get you to do the behavior. The reward doesn't make you do it. You make you do it. So do it. Just leap into it and do it. Then reward yourself. Let your brain figure it out.

Of course some changes won't come easily. But giving up merely guarantees that results won't come at all. Ever.

3. Take radical responsibility

Remember, shame doesn't create change. You're not a bad person. Instead of thinking ill of yourself, use "radical" responsibility to find out how to create the outcomes you want. Deep personal honesty is what's required. You can put it like this: The Easter Bunny didn't make your life the way it is. You did. You may not have understood what you were actually doing at the time you created the life you have now. You may not have been able to predict the outcomes you've gotten through your past choices. But you are the only one who can change what you do now.

The other day I was swimming. It's great exercise and I purposely find a lot of pleasure in it. I practiced the backstroke while looking at a tree so I could stay on course and not swim all over the pool. (I really didn't want to bump other people!) I kept my eye on that tree, and every time I moved out of alignment with the tree, I would change my position so as to come back into alignment.

Lying there in the pool I had a mini-epiphany. The tree moved, or rather, appeared to move, because my alignment was off. Did it move? The truth was that it was my behavior that had resulted in my moving away from the tree. It's not like God or the Unfair Fairy moved the tree! Sometimes we act as if we are doing things perfectly and then, when we don't get the results we wanted, we decide that those results were obviously out of our control. It's as though we think somebody moved our tree while we (with the navigation skills of a Columbus!) were swimming in an absolutely straight line. We are so good at ignoring our actions it's as if our brain is convinced that how we act must remain unassailable in order for us to stay alive!

4. Use Bottom-Up Processing

Often we approach problem-solving by relying on common sense or not tackling our problems until we feel better. Perhaps we think we can "logic" our way out, but then we get stuck, not realizing that logic takes a vacation when fear pops up. When we are unaware of our emotions (time to get mindful!) then we cannot see what's in front of our faces. Remember, your brain will lie to you faster than your body will, so use your body to help your brain "see" better.

Most of your nerves run directionally from the body to the brain, so you have more power if you use your body to influence your brain than if you try to use your brain to influence your body. Try some jumping jacks. Intense physical exercise will usually help you get your brain get back on track.[71]

5. Develop and use Procedural Memory, not just Declarative Memory

Procedural memory is basically habit, like when you brush your teeth before bed. Declarative memory is the stuff that you have to deliberately think about, like the question of which river runs north. If you want to put a behavior into your procedural

> *There will always be some days where no reward feels good enough to get you to do the behavior. The reward doesn't make you do it. You make you do it. So do it.*

---

[71] If it doesn't, maybe it's because you keep thinking the same self-punitive thoughts. More jumping jacks! And quit shoulding all over yourself!

memory you have to practice it over and over.

Here's an example. I have a goal to eat lots of raw vegetables. In order to accomplish this goal I decide on the behavior of eating a big salad for lunch on weekdays. Putting this behavior into procedural memory will make it easier to do in the long run. But first I have to put some effort into practicing both the making and the eating of a big salad for lunch. I do it over and over. I practice finding out how to enjoy it[72]. Once this behavior becomes a habit, I don't have to push myself into it as hard. Doing it takes far less effort.

One the major advantages of creating habits is that procedural memories work even when you are under stress. Declarative memories, on the other hand, don't work so well. When you are anxious, declarative memory is hit hard by that anxiety and you can't rely on logic. So you want to create those habits ahead of time, not on the day of the performance.

Finally, don't think you can skip the work involved in creating these kinds of habits because you are smarter than the average Joe. Knowing more or being smart is no substitute for practicing. You simply must practice— even if you are super smart!

This is Big Idea Number Six, the last Big Idea in the book: *Act yourself into change.*

6. Plan Ahead for Potential Breakdowns

We all run into breakdowns. Sometimes you do your best and obstacles just come up to get in the way of your plans. Often these events

---

[72] For me, pine nuts are the ticket!

> **Big Idea #6:**
>
>   *Act yourself into change. Use your energy to create habits rather than using energy to fuel willpower. Habits are far more efficient.*

cannot be anticipated, but sometimes you can project the most likely events that may sabotage your plans. Instead of falling victim to such circumstances, there are two ways to handle these potential roadblocks. First, try your best to identify all upcoming problems you can imagine. For example, if you'll be busy all weekend, think about how you'll handle mealtimes and exercise during your busy weekend. This way you'll be able to maintain needed balance on your three-legged stool. Second, have general backup plans available for those times when you can't anticipate problems. For example, you could keep a couple protein shakes at work for the times you forget your lunch, or create an alternative exercise plan for when it rains. You won't always be able to prevent future breakdowns, but you'll be ahead of where you might have been otherwise.

7. Find and Replace

Weekends often create kinks in our health plan. Whether it's sleeping in, drinking alcohol, or otherwise letting go of what keeps us sane, you can choose to create new behaviors even when your brain isn't cooperating. For example, if Friday becomes associated with a few beers after work and you know that those few beers lead to sleeping in on Saturday and consequently eating too much sugar and feeling like a blob on Sunday... well, you might want to change that routine. Teach your brain that Friday doesn't have to mean drinking. Friday can mean a lot of things. Then practice those other things over and over until your brain automatically comes up with a variety of associations to Fridays rather than just beer.

Remember, if you kick yourself (and by this I mean doing any self-punitive behavior or any self-criticism) every time you think of beer, your brain will remember that thought more clearly than the message you intend. Then, your efforts will backfire. What you can do instead is this: just notice the tempting thought and then gently turn your mind to another thought. For example, your brain might say, "Friday. Want beer." You can instead say, "Right now I'm mini-golfing. This is nice. Then I'm going for a bike ride. Peace out, brain." If your brain responds like a difficult two year-old, just gently repeat the original message over and over, just as you'd do with a two year-old.

8. Find other pleasures

What else gives you pleasure? Did you know that when you repeatedly indulge in food pleasures, it's harder to find pleasure in other things? This is true for any addiction. Your brain gets hooked on the addiction and then you stop finding as much happiness in other pleasures. To counteract this it helps to plan practice sessions in finding and increasing the pleasures connected to healthy alternatives. Thereby you will create a much richer, more diversified life, which will make it far easier for your brain to make good choices.

9. Want Is Not the Same As Feels Good

The neurotransmitter, dopamine, which is responsible for reminding you how much you want something[cxcii] is not the actual source of the pleasure you feel. It just makes you want to do a fun thing again, whether or not it was in your best interests. It signals entertainment possibilities, not outcome guarantees. For example, you may think you want to eat that pound cake, but after eating it you feel gluggy[73]. It only takes a few minutes after that last bite to feel like a blob, but dopamine won't tell you that blah feeling is an integral part of the pound cake eating outcome. Instead, you have to remember that outcome with the grownup part of your brain.

Remembering that Want is not the same as Actually Feels Good will help you keep your wanting in perspective and reduce its power. Every time you pay attention to dopamine and do what it wants, you simply strengthen your dopamine responses. You actually create more reactivity to the original cue. More reactivity means a bigger dopamine surge of wanting that's even harder to resist. So don't allow the response to happen. The more you practice saying no to dopamine, the more skilled your brain gets at saying no and the easier it becomes.

---

[73]It's a technical term, I know.

10. Take Time For Rituals

In this process of change, make the "want" of dopamine work in your favor! Rituals set off dopamine much more powerfully than non-ritual behavior, so create some healthy, pleasurable rituals around what you really value. You could choose to create rituals about exercise, yoga, sleep, food, religious practice, you name it. Make those rituals special and dopamine will be on *your* side!

You may think you don't enough time to create rituals, much less to do them! Whoa! I urge you to take a hard look at that assumption. You have as much time as you want. We all choose how we allocate our time. Taking time to be calm and deliberate is critically important for your mind-body health. In contrast, continually being in a rush is hard on the relationships in your life. If you persist in your speediness you may find that others have to accommodate to your life rather than having real, connecting relationships with you. If your relationships consist of one-way accommodation, you are missing out, whether or not you are aware of it.

Rituals that motivate and nurture positive change for you could include: a regular family walk after dinner each night, learning some yoga and greeting each day with a sun salutation, enjoying a variety of salads for dinner every Tuesday night, or even getting together with friends for a monthly night out to taste foods from a different culture.

11. Whole-Body Practice Includes Everything!

When you want to make a change, make the change with your whole body. In addition to stepping up on that three-legged stool and letting go of discouraging thoughts, using your whole body includes choosing the way you breathe, choosing your posture, choosing your facial expressions and choosing your voice tone. Don't underestimate the power of these body events on your mind! Simply half-smiling in a gentle way results in increased sensations of happiness.[cxciii] If you experiment, you'll notice a difference in the way you feel when you slump, groaning the words, "I choose health," as compared to when you stand up tall, stretch your arms out, breathe deeply and call out confidently, "I choose health!" Here's another example: if you plan on going to the gym, act like you want to go. Smile at your fellow gym-goers. Let your posture communicate excitement and interest in what you are doing. Just as breathing deeply and extending a firm handshake will diminish anxiety in a job interview, changing your posture, breathing deeply, lifting your facial expressions and thinking kind thoughts about yourself and others will also create more motivation for the health behaviors you are choosing.

12. Respect your boundaries

A boundary is the line that discriminates between things that help you get closer to your goals versus the things that distract you from your goals. A boundary will mean different things to different people, depending on their own personal limits, circumstances and goals. For example, I might find that it crosses the boundary line to answer my telephone after 10 pm. My rationale here is not that I'm trying to be a stick-in-the-mud! It's simply that I've found, through experience, that if I chat after 10 o'clock, I can forget about being calm enough to fall asleep at a time that is best for my body. Sometimes my overall goals make it important to cross that specific line because something more important requires it. But crossing that line frequently when it's not required will only distract me from the outcome I want: getting quality sleep on a regular basis.

If you honor your personal boundaries you will learn to trust yourself.

On the other hand, if you rationalize avoiding doing what your heart tells you to do by calling it a "boundary," you'll feel, deep down, like a fraud.

Respecting your own boundaries will do something wonderful: it will nurture and enlarge your motivation. But when you ignore your essential needs over and over, you will allow discouragement to erode your motivation. You start to distrust yourself, your thoughts, your feelings, even your wisdom.

I have a really fun client named, oh, let's say Andromeda. Andromeda had zero motivation to do anything when she first came to see me. She also had no conception of a boundary. She let people make decisions for her, even when she was dreadfully unhappy about the outcomes. She had no limits for herself. Her sleeping, eating and shopping were based on whatever she felt like at the moment. She had grown up in a authoritarian home where obedience was paramount. She was overrun by others who told her what to do at her job, and as a result, she indulged every whim that came into her head in her personal life, attempting to create some balance between her independence and others' demands. The results she had were that she was spending a ton of money on things she didn't want and she felt physically rotten. Furthermore, she would practically vomit at the thought of being asked to do anything!

She and I worked on learning about boundaries to help her take better care of herself. After she saw that others would actually respect her needs when she presented them skillfully, she started creating some boundaries for herself. But these personal boundaries took longer to solidify because she would often get stuck in the idea that she deserved to indulge herself due to her painful history. The indulgences never led to long-term happiness, and most of the time, any one pleasure was extremely short-lived.

One of the coolest things she found in this journey was a resurrection of her motivation. She started to feel alive again. She even started to connect to others in a way that reduced her painful loneliness and increased a sense of self-efficacy. She let others see the star within.

Respecting your boundaries (with others and with yourself[74]) strengthens your motivation because you feel more human, alive, and powerful.

Conclusion

You've reached the end of this book.

Here's the part where you can jump up and down, foaming at the mouth for change, the place

---

[74] Boundaries with yourself are what I call self-discipline.

in the book where you are screaming "Now! I want to start now!"

No? Okay, so that was a fantasy on my part. Well, I'm going to let you in on a little secret: That's not even what I want from you. The truth is that lasting change isn't a result of being in a frenzy of Want. It's something solid that happens because you work on it every day—without relying on feeling motivated in order to get started. It's about choosing to be grown-up in your body and your brain.

So get started, whether or not you are motivated, whether or not you are happy, and whether or not you feel up to it. Act yourself into change. Just begin.

Remember — the old saying: The best time to plant an oak tree is 20 years ago. The next best time is today.

Start today.

I'd love to hear how it goes.[75]

---

[75] You can email me at dr.alison@caldwellandrews.com or check out my website: mindbodytotalhealth.com

Acknowledgements

If it weren't for Mack Stephenson, this book would not have been written. Thank you, Mack. You are a dear friend and interacting with you has made me a better person.

If it weren't for Greg Halliday, Mack wouldn't have talked to me about writing this book. Thank you, Greg. You are a total inspiration. I was thinking about you when I talked about people who seem superhuman.

My deepest thanks to my family who put up with all the chaos involved as I worked to finish this book. You're the best. Ever.

And to my remarkable mother, Anita Osmond, who indefatigably, scrupulously and effectively edited for me! Without her tender loving care, the book would be far, far less readable.

I also received very helpful, thorough editing from Caitlin Weeks, English Graduate Extraordinaire. Of the much valuable help she gave me, nothing was more appreciated than her willingness to do a mind-breaking review of all of the references and formatting.

Other great comments and edits were suggested by Brandon Kreutzkamp, whose help in deciphering Irritable Bowel Syndrome was invaluable; by Russ Osmond, who inspired structure, reminded me to stay on task and keep it simple; by Cynthia Nielsen who provided wonderful edits, by Cecily Hart who saved me from a few grave errors (well, I might not literally have died); from John Andrews and from Natalie Dark.

When I first saw the cover that Kendall Bird designed it filled my heart. Thank you, Kendall, for being such a true artist that you read my soul.

Finally, thank you most especially to my dear patients whose struggles bring light to every dark place. I have learned much from you and look forward to a bright future!

INDEX

REFERENCES

[1]Gerber MA, Baltimore RS, Eaton CB, Gewitz M, Rowley AH, Shulman ST, Taubert KA. "Prevention of rheumatic fever and diagnosis and treatment of acute streptococcal pharyngitis." *AHA Scientific Statement.* Circulation 2009; 119: 1541-1551.

[2]ibid

[3]Choby BA. "Diagnosis and treatment of streptococcal pharyngitis." *Am Fam Physician.* 2009 Mar 1;79(5):383-390.

[4]Chin, TK. "Pediatric rheumatic fever." *Medscape Reference.* 2010 (Feb 25). Available at http://emedicine.medscape.com/article/1007946-overview. Accessed February 25, 2012.

[5]Newman DH. "Antibiotics for strep do more harm than good." *Emergency Physicians Monthly* (online magazine). Available at: http://www.epmonthly.com/columns/in-my-opinion/antibiotics. Accessed February 28, 2012.

[6]Choby BA. "Diagnosis and Treatment of Streptococcal Pharyngitis." *Am Fam Physician.* 2009 Mar 1;79(5):383-390.

[7]Parillo SJ, Parillo CV. "Rheumatic Fever in Emergency Medicine." *Medscape Reference.* 2010 (March 23). Available at :http://emedicine.medscape.com/article/808945-overview#showall Accessed February 11, 2012.

[8]Newman DH. Antibiotics for strep do more harm than good.*Emergency Physicians Monthly* (online magazine). Available at: http://www.epmonthly.com/columns/in-my-opinion/antibiotics. Accessed February 28, 2012.

[9]ibid.

[10]Siri-Tarino PW, Sun Q, Hu FB, Krauss RM. "Meta-analysis of prospective cohort studies evaluating the association of saturated fat with cardiovascular disease." *Am J Clin Nutr* March 2010 vol. 91 no. 3 535-546

[11] Edelson M, Sharot T, Dolan RJ, Yadin D. (2011, Jul 1). Following the crowd: brain substrates of long-term memory conformity. *Science.* Vol. 333(6038), 108-111

[12]Dwairy M, Dowell AC, Stahl JC. (2011, Aug 23). The application of foraging theory to the information searching behaviour of general practitioners. *BMC Fam Pract* 23, 12:90.

[13]Hoogendam A, Stalenhoef AF, Robbé PF, Overbeke AJ. (2008, Oct 3). Answers to questions posed during daily patient care are more likely to be answered by UpToDate than PubMed. *J Med Internet Res.* 10(4), e29.

[14]Sánchez-Villegas A, Delgado-Rodríguez M, Alonso A, et al. (2009). Association of the Mediterranean dietary pattern with the incidence of depression: the Seguimiento Universidad de Navarra/University of Navarra follow-up (SUN) cohort. *Arch*

Gen Psychiatry. 66, 1090-1098.

[15]Amminger GP, Schäfer MR, Papageorgiou K, et al. (2010). Long-chain omega-3 fatty acids for indicated prevention of psychotic disorders: a randomized, placebo-controlled trial. *Arch Gen Psychiatry.* 67, 146-154. *and*

Judge MP, Beck CT, Durham H, et al. (2011). Maternal docosahexaenoic acid (DHA, 22:6n-3) consumption during pregnancy decreases postpartum depression (PPD) symptomatology. *FASEB J* 25, 349.7.

[16] Effects of dietary coconut oil on the biochemical and anthropometric profiles of women presenting abdominal obesity. Lipids. 2009 Jul;44(7):593-601.

[17]Mursu J, Robien K, Harnack LJ, Park K, Jacobs DR Jr. (2011, Oct 10). Dietary supplements and mortality rate in older women: the Iowa Women's Health Study. *Arch Intern Med.* 171(18), 1625-33.

[18]Mursu J, Robien K, Harnack LJ, Park K, Jacobs DR Jr. (2011, Oct 10). Dietary supplements and mortality rate in older women: the Iowa Women's Health Study. *Arch Intern Med* 171(18), 1625-33.

[19] Bushman BJ, Baumeister RF, Stack AD. Catharsis, aggression, and persuasive influence: self-fulfilling or self-defeating prophecies? *J Pers Soc Psychol.* 1999 Mar;76(3):367-76.

[20] Zhong CB, DeVoe SE. You Are How You Eat: Fast Food and Impatience. *Psychological Science* May 2010 vol. 21 no. 5 619-622

[21]Beezhold BL, Johnston CS, Daigle DR. (2010). Vegetarian diets are associated with healthy mood states: a cross-sectional study in Seventh Day Adventist adults. *Nutr J.* 9, 26.

[22]Beezhold BL, Johnston CS. (2012). Restriction of meat, fish, and poultry in omnivores improves mood: A pilot randomized controlled trial. *Nutr J.* 11, 9.

[23] Schmid KM, Ohlrogge JB. Lipid metabolism in plants. In Vance DE, Vance JE (Eds). *Biochemistry of lipids, lipoproteins and membranes*, 4th ed., Elsevier Science (p 93).

[24] Young VR, Bier DM, Pellet PL. A theoretical basis for increasing current estimates of the amino acid requirements in adult man, with experimental support. *Am J Clin Nutr.* 1989 Jul;50(1):80-92.

Young VR, Bier DM, Pellett PL.

[25] Fushiki, Kawai. (2003). Chemical reception of fats in the oral cavity and the mechanism of addiction to dietary fat. *Chemical Sense.* 30(1), i184-i185.

[26] Fushiki, Kawai. (2003). Chemical reception of fats in the oral cavity and the mechanism of addiction to dietary fat. Chemical Sense. 30(1), i184-i185.

[27·] Stratford JM, Contreras RJ. (2010). Peripheral gustatory processing of free fatty acids. In Montmayeur JM and le Coutre

J (Eds), *Fat detection: Taste, texture, and post ingestive effects.* (pp. 123-136) Boca Raton:FL.

28 Astrup A, Dyerberg J, Elwood P, Hermansen K, Hu FB, Jakobsen MU, Kok FJ, Krauss RM, Lecerf JM, LeGrand P, et al. The role of reducing intakes of saturated fat in the prevention of cardiovascular disease: Where does the evidence stand in 2010? *Am J Clin Nutr* 2011;93: 684–8.

29 Dulloo AG, Fathi M, Mensi N, Girardier L. Twenty-four-hour energy expenditure and urinary catecholamines of humans consuming low-to-moderate amounts of medium-chain triglycerides: A dose-response study in a human respiratory chamber. *Eur J Clin Nutr.* 1996 Mar;50(3):152-8.

30 Kluger J. (2013, Jul 25). How the moon messes with your sleep. *Time: Science and Space.* Retrieved from http://science.time.com/2013/07/25/how-the-moon-messes-with-your-sleep/

31 Srinivasan V, Mohamed M, Kato H. (2012, Jan). Melatonin in bacterial and viral infections with focus on sepsis: A review. *Pub Med,* 6(1), 30-90. Retrieved from http://www.ncbi.nlm.nih.gov/pubmed/22264213

32 Bubenik GA, Blask DE, Brown GM, Maestroni GJ, Pang SF, Reiter RJ, Viswanathan M, Zisapel N. (1998). Prospects of the clinical utilization of melatonin. *Pub Med,* 7(4), 195-219. Retrieved from http://www.ncbi.nlm.nih.gov/pubmed/9730580

33 Huber R, Hill SL, Holladay C, Biesiadecki M, Tononi G, Cirelli C. (2005). Sleep homeostasis in drosophila melanogaster. *Sleep* 27(4), 628–639.

34 National Institutes of Health. (2011). *Your guide to healthy sleep.* Retrieved from http://www.nhlbi.nih.gov/health/public/sleep/healthy_sleep.pdf

35 O'Donnell E. (2010). Lost sleep is hard to find. *Harvard Magazine,* Retrieved from http://harvardmagazine.com/2010/07/lost-sleep-is-hard-to-find

36 Stickgold R. (2005, Oct). Sleep-dependent memory consolidation. *Nature,* 437, 1272-1278

37 Bellesi M, Pfister-Genskow MP, Maret S, Keles S, Tononi G, Cirelli C. Effects of Sleep and Wake on Oligodendrocytes and Their Precursors. *The Journal of Neuroscience,* 4 September 2013, 33(36):14288-14300.

38 King CR, Knutson KL, Rathouz PJ, Sidney S, Liu K, Lauderdale DS. (2008, Dec 24). Short sleep duration and incident coronary artery calcification. *JAMA.* 300(24), 2859-66.

39 Sleep 2010, the 24th annual meeting of the Associated Professional Sleep Societies LLC, June 7, 2010, San Antonio, Texas.

40 Hefferenan M. (2013). THE DANGERS OF "WILLFUL

BLINDNESS." Retrieved from http://www.ted.com/talks/
margaret_heffernan_the_dangers_of_willful_blindness.html

[41] J. R. Pleis et al. (2010). Summary health statistics for US
adults: National health interview survey, 2009. Conducted by
the Centers for Disease Control and Prevention, U.S.
Department of Health and Human Services/National Center for
Health Statistics, , 10 (249).

[42] Joseph Ciccolo et al. (2011). Resistance training as an aid to
standard smoking cessation treatment: A pilot study. *Nicotine
and Tobacco Research.* 13(8), 756-760.

[43] Ratey J. (2008) Spark: The Revolutionary New Science of
Exercise and the Brain. New York: Little, Brown and Company.
p. 245

[44] Ratey J. (2008) *Spark: The Revolutionary New Science of
Exercise and the Brain.* New York: Little, Brown and Company.

[45] Merritt R. (2000 Sept. 22). Study: Exercise has long-lasting
effect on depression. *Duke Today.* Retrieved from
http://today.duke.edu/2000/09/exercise922.html

[46] artinowich K, Lu B. Interaction between BDNF and Serotonin:
Role in Mood Disorders. *Neuropsychopharmacology Reviews*
(2008) 33, 73–83; doi:10.1038/sj.npp.1301571; published
online 19 September 2007

[47] Rimer J, Dwan K, Lawlor DA, Greig CA, McMurdo M, Morley W,
Mead GE. (2012, Jul.) Exercise for depression.
Cochrane Database Syst Rev. 11(7).

[48] http://summaries.cochrane.org/CD004366/exercise-for-
depression. Retrieved 10/10/2013.

[49] Warner-Schmidt JL, Duman RS. (2006). Hippocampal
neurogenesis: Opposing effects of stress and antidepressant
treatment. *Hippocampus* 16(3), 239-49.

[50] Broman-Fulks, J. J., Berman, M. E., Rabian, B., & Webster, M.
J. (2004). Effects of aerobic exercise on anxiety sensitivity.
Behaviour Research and Therapy, 42(2): 125-136.

[51] Ratey J. (2008) *Spark: The Revolutionary New Science of
Exercise and the Brain.* New York: Little, Brown and Company.

[52] Winter,B., Breitenstein, C., Mooren, F.C., Voelker, K., Fobkes,
M., et al. (2007). High impact running improves learning.
Neurobiology of Learning and Memory. 87(4), 597-609

[53] Masley S, Roetzheim R, Gualtieri T. (2009, Jun.). Aerobic
exercise enhances cognitive flexibility. *J Clin Psychol Med
Settings.* 16(2),186-93.

[54] Ratey J. (2008)*Spark: The Revolutionary New Science of Exercise
and the Brain.* New York: Little, Brown and Company

[55] Cohen, G., Shamus, E. (2009 Apr.) Depressed, low self-esteem:
What can exercise do for you? *The Internet Journal of Allied
Health Sciences and Practice.* 7(2). Retrieved from
http://ijahsp.nova.edu/articles/Vol7Num2/cohen.htm

Malhotra R., Bradshaw DH., The effect of exercise walking on cortisol levels in patients with fibromyalgia. *PDFIO*. Retrieved from http://www.pdfio.com/k-6311811.html# Georgia State University. (1998 Mar, 4) Aerobic exercise main page. Gsu.edu. Retrieved 09/14/2013 from http://www2.gsu.edu/~wwwfit/aerobice.html

56 Constance G. Bacon et al.. (2003). Sexual function in men older than 50 years of age. *Annals of Internal Medicine*. 139(3), 161-168.

57 Ratey J. (2008) *Spark: The Revolutionary New Science of Exercise and the Brain*. New York: Little, Brown and Company

58 Naci H, Ioannidis JP. Comparative effectiveness of exercise and drug interventions on mortality outcomes: metaepidemiological study. *BMJ 2013;347:f5577*

59 http://www.bloomberg.com/news/2013-10-01/exercise-may-be-as-effective-as-drugs-in-treating-heart-disease.html

60 Alberts B, Johnson A, Lewis J, et al. Molecular Biology of the Cell. 4th edition. New York: Garland Science; 2002. Blood Vessels and Endothelial Cells. Available from: http://www.ncbi.nlm.nih.gov/books/NBK26848/. Accessed 12 Oct 2013.

61 Blake GJ, Ridker PM. (2011). Are statins anti-inflammatory? *Curr Control Trials Cardiovasc Med*. 1(3), 161–165. Retrieved from http://www.ncbi.nlm.nih.gov/pmc/articles/PMC59622/

62 Fujiwara N, Kobayashi K. (2005, Jun.) Macrophages in inflammation. *Curr Drug Targets Inflamm Allergy*. 4(3), 281-6.

63 St.Charles A. Inflammation: causes, prevention & control. *INR Health Update*, Feb 2011.

64 (2012, Sept.). Knee injections offer minimal relief from arthritis pain. *HarvMens Health Watch*. 17(2), 8.

65 Choi HK, Curhan G. (2008, Feb.). Soft drinks, fructose consumption, and the risk of gout in men: prospective cohort study
BMJ 336(7639), 309-312.

66 Grimstvedt ME, Woolf K, Milliron BJ, Manore MM. (2010, Aug.) Lower healthy eating index – 2005 dietary quality scores in older women with rheumatoid arthritis v. healthy controls. *Public Health Nutr*. 13(8), 1170-7. Retrieved from http://www.ncbi.nlm.nih.gov/pubmed/20188003

67 Christensen LP.(2009, Jan.).Galactolipids as potential health promoting compounds in vegetable foods.*Recent Pat Food NutrAgric* 1(1), 50-8.

68 Cohen S, Janicki-Deverts D, Doyle WJ, Miller GE, Frank E, Rabin BS, Turner RB. Chronic stress, glucocorticoid receptor resistance, inflammation, and disease risk PNAS 2012 109 (16) 5995-5999; published ahead of print April 2, 2012, doi:10.1073/pnas.1118355109. Accessed Oct. 11, 2013.

69 Ley, R.E. (2010). Obesity and the human microbiome. *Curr Opin Gastroenterology*. 26(1), 5-11.

[70]Mariat, D., Firmesse, O., Levenez, F., Guimaraes, V.D., Sokol, H., Dore, J., Corthier, G., Furet, J.P. (2009, Jun). The Firmicutes/Bacteroidetes ratio of the human microbiota changes with age. *BMC Microbiology.* 9(123)

[71]Ley, R.E. (2010).Obesity and the human microbiome. *CurrOpin Gastroenterology.*26(1), 5-11.

[72]DiBaise, J.K., Zhang, H., Crowell, M.D., Krajmalnik-Brown, R., Anton Decker, G., Rittmann, B.E. (2008, Apr.). Gut microbiota and its possible relationship with obesity.*Mayo Foundation for Medical Education and Research.* 83(4),460-469.

[73]Ley, R.E. (2010).Obesity and the human microbiome.*CurrOpin Gastroenterology.*26(1), 5-11.

[74]Duncan, S.H., Belenguer, A., Holtrop, G., Johnstone, A.M., Flint, H.J., Lobley, G.E. (2007, Feb.). Reduced Dietary Intake of Carbohydrates by Obese Subjects Results in Decreased Concentrations of Butyrate and Butyrate-Producing Bacteria in Feces. *Appl Environ Microbiol.*, 73(4), 1073-1078

[75]Le Chatelier E., et al. Richness of human gut microbiome correlates with metabolic markers. *Nature.* 2013 Aug 29;500(7464):541-6.

[76] Cotillard, A., et al. *Nature.* 2013 Aug 29;500(7464):585-8. doi: 10.1038/nature12480.

[77] Peterson CA, Heffernan ME. Serum tumor necrosis factor-alpha concentrations are negatively correlated with serum 25(OH)D concentrations in healthy women.*J Inflamm*(Lond). 2008 Jul 24;5:10. doi: 10.1186/1476-9255-5-10.

[78] Hansson GK. Inflammation, Atherosclerosis, and Coronary Artery Disease. N Engl J Med 2005; 352:1685-169

[79] Alberts B, Johnson A, Lewis J, et al. Molecular Biology of the Cell. 4th edition. New York: Garland Science; 2002. Blood Vessels and Endothelial Cells. Available from: http://www.ncbi.nlm.nih.gov/books/NBK26848. Accessed 12Oct2013.

[80] Sachdeva A, Cannon CP, Deedwania PC, LaBresh KA, Smith SC, Dai D, Hernandez A, Fonarow G. (2009, Jan). Lipid levels in patients hospitalized with coronary artery disease: An analysis of 136,905 hospitalizations in Get With The Guidelines. *American Heart Journal* 157(1), 111-117.

[81] Schupf N, Costa R, Luchsinger J, Tang MX, Lee JH, Mayeux R. (2005, Feb). Relationship between plasma lipids and all-cause mortality in nondemented elderly. *J Am Geriatr Soc.*53(2), 219-26.

[82] ibid

[83] Brotons C. (1990). Reducing cholesterol levels in elderly persons. *JAMA.* 263(21), 2889-2890

[84] Winawer SJ, Flehinger BJ, Buchalter J, Herbert E, Shike M. Declining. (1990). serum cholesterol levels prior to diagnosis of colon cancer: A time-trend, case-control study. *JAMA.* 263(15),

2083-2085.

[85] Behar S, Graff E, Reicher-Reiss H, Boyko V, Benderly M, Shotan A, Brunner D. (1997, Jan). Low total cholesterol is associated with high total mortality in patients with coronary heart disease. The Bezafibrate Infarction Prevention (BIP) Study Group. *Eur Heart J*.18(1), 52-9.

[86] Saini R, Saini S, Sharma S. Potential of probiotics in controlling cardiovascular diseases. *J Cardiovasc Dis Res*. 2010 Oct-Dec; 1(4): 213–214.

[87] Holvoet P, Theilmeier G, Shivalkar B, Flameng W, Collen D. LDL hypercholesterolemia is associated with accumulation of oxidized LDL, atherosclerotic plaque growth, and compensatory vessel enlargement in coronary arteries of miniature pigs.Arterioscler Thromb Vasc Biol. 1998 Mar;18(3):415-22.

[88] Guyton JR. Atherosclerosis - a story of cells, cholesterol and clots. Available at http://classes.biology.ucsd.edu/bisp194-2.WI11/Guyton%20article.pdf. Accessed 14 Oct 2013.

[89] Boaventura BC, Di Pietro PF, Stefanuto A, Klein GA, de Morais EC, de Andrade F, Wazlawik E, da Silva EL. (2012, Jun). Association of mate tea (Ilex paraguariensis) intake and dietary intervention and effects on oxidative stress biomarkers of dyslipidemic subjects. *Nutrition*. 28(6), 657-64.

[90] *The American Journal of Clinical Nutrition*(2004, Oct) 23(5), 501S-5055

[91] Journal American College Nutrition (2004). 23,501, 05S.

[92] Nouwen A, Nefs G, Caramlau I, Connock M, Winkley K, Lloyd CE, Peyrot M, Pouwer F; European Depression in Diabetes Research Consortium.Prevalence of depression in individuals with impaired glucose metabolism or undiagnosed diabetes: a systematic review and meta-analysis of the European Depression in Diabetes (EDID) Research Consortium. Diabetes Care. 2011 Mar;34(3):752-62. Review.

[93] Katon, WJ. (2011) Epidemiology and treatment of depression in patients with chronic medical illness. Dialogues in Clinical Neuroscience, 13, 1 (7-23).

[94] Knol M, Twisk J, Beekman A, Heine R, Snoek F, Pouwer F. Depression as a risk factor for the onset of type 2 diabetes: a meta-analysis. DIABETOLOGIA 49:837-845, 2006.

[95] Mezuk B, Eaton WW, Albrecht S, Golden SH. Depression and type 2 diabetes over the lifespan. Diabetes Care 31:2383-2390, 2008.

[96] Engum A. The role of depression and anxiety in onset of diabetes in a large population-based study. J Psychosom Res 62:31-38, 2007.

[97] Gois C, Barbosa A, Ferro A, Santos AL, Sousa F, Akiskal H, Akiskal K, Figueira ML. The role of affective temperaments in metabolic control in patients with type 2 diabetes. J Affect Disord. 2011 Nov;134(1-3):52-8. Epub 2011 Jun 8.

[98] Bjorntorp P (2001) Do stress reactions cause abdominal obesity

and comorbidities? Obes Rev 2:73–86

[99]Faulenbach H, Uthoff K, Schwegler G. A., Spinas C., Schmid P., Wiesli M. Effect of psychological stress on glucose control in patients with Type 2 diabetes

[100]Biol Psychol. 2011 May;87(2):234-40. Epub 2011 Mar 16

[101]Weber-Hamann B, Hentschel F, Kniest A et al (2002) Hypercortisolemic depression is associated with increased intra-abdominal fat. Psychosom Med 64:274–277. Also see: Bjorntorp P, Holm G, Rosmond R (1999) Hypothalamic arousal, insulin resistance and type 2 diabetes mellitus. Diabet Med 16:373–383

[102]Kawakami N, Araki S, Takatsuka N, Shimizu H, Ishibashi H. Overtime, psychosocial work conditions, and occurance of non-insulin dependent diabetes mellitus in Japanes men. J EPIDEMIOL COMMUNITY HEALTH 53:359-363, 1999.

[103]Melamed S, Shirom A, Toker S, Shapira I. Burnout and risk of type 2 diabetes: a prospective study of apparently healthy employed persons. PSYCHOSOM MED 68:863-869, 2006.

[104]Norberg N, Stenlund H, Lindahl B, Andersson C, Eriksson JW, Weinehall. Work stress and low emotional support is associated with increased risk of future type 2 diabetes in women. DIABETES RES CLIN PRACT 76:368-377, 2007.

[105]Nowotny B, Cavka M, Herder C, Löffler H, Poschen U, Joksimovic L et al. Effects of acute psychological stress on glucose metabolism and subclinical inflammation in patients with post-traumatic stress disorder. Horm Metab Res 2010; 42: 746-753.

[106]http://articles.mercola.com/sites/articles/archive/2009/03/2 6/The-Little-Known-Secrets-about-Bleached-Flour.aspx Accessed 14Oct2013.

[107]Results of longitudinal studies suggest that not only depression but also general emotional stress and anxiety, sleeping problems, anger, and hostility are associated with an increased risk for the development of type 2 diabetes." (Does Emotional Stress Cause Type 2 Diabetes Mellitus? A Review from the European Depression in Diabetes (EDID) Research Consortium)

[108] Panwar H, Rashmi HM, Batish VK, Grover S. Probiotics as potential biotherapeutics in the management of type 2 diabetes - prospects and perspectives. *Diabetes Metab Res Rev.* 2013 Feb;29(2):103-12. doi: 10.1002/dmrr.2376.

[109] Christakos S, Hewison M, Gardner DG, Wagner CL, Sergeev IN, Rutten E, Pittas AG, Boland R, Ferrucci L. Vitamin D beyond bone. Ann N Y Acad Sci. 2013;11:45–58. doi: 10.1111/nyas.12129

[110]Stetler C, Miller GE. Depression and hypothalamic-pituitary-adrenal activation: a quantitative summary of four decades of research. Psychosom Med. 2011 Feb-Mar;73(2):114-26. Epub

2011 Jan 21.

[111]Bravo JA, Forsythe P, Chew MV, Escaravage E, Savignac HM, Dinan TG, Bienenstock J, Cryan JF. Ingestion of Lactobacillus strain regulates emotional behavior and central GABA receptor expression in a mouse via the vagus nerve. Proc Natl Acad Sci U S A. 2011 Sep 20;108(38):16050-5. Epub 2011 Aug 29.

[112]Bowe WP, Logan AC. Acne vulgaris, probiotics and the gut-brain-skin axis - back to the future? Gut Pathog. 2011 Jan 31;3(1):1.

[113] Wilkins, Consuelo H. M.D.; Sheline, Yvette I. M.D.; Roe, Catherine M. Ph.D.; Birge, Stanley J. M.D.; Morris, John C. M.D. Vitamin D Deficiency Is Associated With Low Mood and Worse Cognitive Performance in Older Adults. American Journal of Geriatric Psychiatry: December 2006 - Volume 14 - Issue 12 - pp 1032-1040

[114] http://www.uptodate.com/contents/vitamin-d-deficiency-beyond-the-basics. Accessed 14 Oct 2013.

[115] Diamond T, Wong YK, Golombick T. Effect of oral cholecalciferol 2,000 versus 5,000 IU on serum vitamin D, PTH, bone and muscle strength in patients with vitamin D deficiency. Osteoporos Int. 2012 Mar 16.

[116]Rubin, M. G., Kim, K., & Logan, A. C. (2008). Acne vulgaris, mental health, and omega-3 fatty acids: A report of cases. Lipids in Health and Disease, 7, 36

[117]Kiecolt-Glaser, J. K., Belury, M.A., Porter, K., Beversdoft, D., Lemeshow, S., & Glaser, R. (2007). Depressive symptoms, omega-6: omega-3 fatty acids, and inflammation in older adults. Psychosomatic Medicine, 69, 217-224.

[118]Logan, A. C. (2004). Omega-3 fatty acids and major depression: A primer for the mental health professional. Lipids in Health and Disease, 3, 25

[119]Peet, M., & Stokes, C. (2005). Omega-3 fatty acids in the treatment of psychiatric disorders. Drugs, 65, 1051-1059.

[120]Logan, A. C. (2004). Omega-3 fatty acids and major depression: A primer for the mental health professional. Lipids in Health and Disease, 3, 25

[121]Kiecolt-Glaser JK, Belury MA, Andridge R, Malarkey WB, Glaser R. Omega-3 supplementation lowers inflammation and anxiety in medical students: a randomized controlled trial. Brain Behav Immun. 2011 Nov;25(8):1725-34. Epub 2011 Jul 19.

[122] Kiecolt-Glaser, J. K., Belury, M.A., Porter, K., Beversdoft, D., Lemeshow, S., & Glaser, R. (2007). Depressive symptoms, omega-6: omega-3 fatty acids, and inflammation in older adults. Psychosomatic Medicine, 69, 217-224.

[123]Peet, M., & Stokes, C. (2005). Omega-3 fatty acids in the treatment of psychiatric disorders. Drugs, 65, 1051-1059.

[124]Harvey AG. 2011 Sleep and circadian functioning: critical mechanisms in the mood disorders? Annu Rev Clin Psychol. Apr;7:297-319.

[125]Cho HJ, Lavretsky H, Olmstead R, Levin MJ, Oxman MN, Irwin MR. 2008. Sleep disturbance and depression recurrence in community-dwelling older adults: a prospective study. Am. J. Psychiatry 165:1534–50

[126]Reynolds CF 3rd, Frank E, Houck PR, Mazumdar S, Dew MA, et al. 1997. Which elderly patients with remitted depression remain well with continued interpersonal psychotherapy after discontinuation of antidepressant medication? Am. J. Psychiatry 154:958–62

[127]J.A. Blumenthal and M.A. Babyak, et al. Exercise and pharmacotherapy in the treatment of major depressive disorder. Psychosom. Med., 69 7 (2007), pp. 587–596.

[128] Hoffman BM, Babyak MA, Craighead WE, Sherwood A, Doraiswamy PM, Coons MJ, Blumenthal JA. Exercise and pharmacotherapy in patients with major depression: one-year follow-up of the SMILE study. Psychosom Med. 2011 Feb-Mar;73(2):127-33. Epub 2010 Dec 10.

[129]Eyre H, Baune BT. Neuroimmunological effects of physical exercise in depression. Brain, Behavior, and Immunity, Available online 2 October 2011, ISSN 0889-1591, 10.1016/j.bbi.2011.09.015.

[130]Milaneschi Y, Bandinelli S, Penninx BW, Corsi AM, Lauretani F, Vazzana R, Semba RD, Guralnik JM, Ferrucci L.The relationship between plasma carotenoids and depressive symptoms in older persons.World J Biol Psychiatry. 2011 Sep 20. [Epub ahead of print]

[131].a) Dowlati Y, Herrmann N, Swardfager W, et al. A meta-analysis of cytokines in major depression. Biol Psychiatry. 2010;67:446–57.
b) Howren MB, Lamkin DM, Suls J. Associations of depression with C-reactive protein, IL-1, and IL-6: a meta-analysis. Psychosom Med. 2009;71:171–86.
c) Zorilla E, Luborsky L, McKay J, et al. The relationship of depression and stressors to immunological assays: a meta-analytic review. Brain Behav Immun. 2001;15:199–226.

[132]Lotrich FE, El-Gabalawy H, Guenther LC, Ware CF. 2011. The role of inflammation in the pathophysiology of depression: different treatments and their effects. J Rheumatol Suppl. 2011 Nov;88:48-54.

[133]Haroon E, Raison CL, Miller AH.Neuropsychopharmacology. Psychoneuroimmunology Meets Neuropsychopharmacology: Translational Implications of the Impact of Inflammation on Behavior. 2011 Sep 14. doi: 10.1038/npp.2011.205. [Epub ahead of print]

[134]Christmas DM, Potokar J, Davies SJ.Neuropsychiatr Dis Treat. A biological pathway linking inflammation and depression: activation of indoleamine 2,3-dioxygenase.2011;7:431-9. Epub 2011 Jul 13.

135Capuron L, Gumnick JF, Musselman DL, et al. Neurobehavioral effects of interferon-alpha in cancer patients: phenomenology and paroxetine responsiveness of symptom dimensions. Neuropsychopharmacol. 2002;26:643–52.

136Raison CL, Miller AH. Is Depression an Inflammatory Disorder? Current Psychiatry Reports (2011) 13:6, 467-475.

137 Irwin MR, Wang M, Campomayor CO, Collado-Hidalgo A, Cole S. 2006. Sleep deprivation and activation of morning levels of cellular and genomic markers of inflammation.Arch Intern Med. Sep 18;166(16):1756-62.

138 Gleeson M, Bishop NC, Stensel DJ, Lindley MR, Mastana SS, Nimmo MA. 2011. The anti-inflammatory effects of exercise: mechanisms and implications for the prevention and treatment of disease. Nat Rev Immunol. 2011 Aug 5;11(9):607-15.

139Copeland WE, Shanahan L, Worthman C, Angold A, Costello EJ.2012. Cumulative depression episodes predict later C-reactive protein levels: a prospective analysis. Biol Psychiatry. 2012 Jan 1;71(1):15-21. Epub 2011 Nov 1.

140Kupper N, Widdershoven JW, Pedersen SS. 2011 Cognitive/affective and somatic/affective symptom dimensions of depression are associated with current and future inflammation in heart failure patients. J Affect Disord. Nov 29. 2011.

141 Kiecolt-Glaser JK.Stress, food, and inflammation: psychoneuroimmunology and nutrition at the cutting edge.Psychosom Med. 2010 May;72(4):365-9. Epub 2010 Apr 21.

142 Feher J, Jovacs I, Balacco G. Role of gastrointestinal inflammations in the development and treatment of depression. Orv Hetil. 2011 Sep 11;152(37):1477-85.

143 Bar M. A cognitive neuroscience hypothesis of mood and depression. Trends Cogn Sci. 2009 Nov;13(11):456-63. Epub 2009

144 O'Malley D, Quigley EM, Dinan TG, Cryan JF. Do interactions between stress and immune responses lead to symptom exacerbations in irritable bowel syndrome? Brain Behav Immun. 2011 Oct;25(7):1333-41. Epub 2011 Apr 23.

145Okami Y, Kato T, Nin G, Harada K, Aoi W, Wada S, Higashi A, Okuyama Y, Takakuwa S, Ichikawa H, Kanazawa M, FukudoS.Lifestyle and psychological factors related to irritable bowel syndrome in nursing and medical school students. J Gastroenterol. 2011 Dec;46(12):1403-10. Epub 2011 Aug 24.

146 O'Malley D, Quigley EM, Dinan TG, Cryan JF. Do interactions between stress and immune responses lead to symptom exacerbations in irritable bowel syndrome? Brain Behav Immun. 2011 Oct;25(7):1333-41. Epub 2011 Apr 23.

147Spiller, RC. Potential future therapies for Irritable Bowel Syndrome: Will Disease Modifying Therapy as Opposed to Symptomatic Control Become a Reality? GastroenterolClin N

Am 34 (2005) 337–354

[148]Okami Y, Kato T, Nin G, Harada K, Aoi W, Wada S, Higashi A, Okuyama Y, Takakuwa S, Ichikawa H, Kanazawa M, FukudoS.Lifestyle and psychological factors related to irritable bowel syndrome in nursing and medical school students. J Gastroenterol. 2011 Dec;46(12):1403-10. Epub 2011 Aug 24.

[149]Hertig VL, Cain KC, Jarrett ME, Burr RL, HeitkemperMM.Daily stress and gastrointestinal symptoms in women with irritable bowel syndrome.

[150]Faresjö A, Grodzinsky E, Johansson S, WallanderMA, Timpka T, AkerlindI.Eur Psychosocial factors at work and in every day life are associated with irritable bowel syndrome. J Epidemiol. 2007;22(7):473-80. Epub 2007 May 5.

[151] O'Malley D, Quigley EM, Dinan TG, Cryan JF. Do interactions between stress and immune responses lead to symptom exacerbations in irritable bowel syndrome? Brain Behav Immun. 2011 Oct;25(7):1333-41. Epub 2011 Apr 23.

[152] O'Malley D, Quigley EM, Dinan TG, Cryan JF. Do interactions between stress and immune responses lead to symptom exacerbations in irritable bowel syndrome? Brain Behav Immun. 2011 Oct;25(7):1333-41. Epub 2011 Apr 23.

[153]Bradford K, Shih W, Videlock E, Presson AP, Naliboff BD, Mayer EA, Chang L. Association between Early Adverse Life Events and Irritable Bowel Syndrome.ClinGastroenterolHepatol. 2011 Dec 15. [Epub ahead of print]

[154]Bradford K, Shih W, Videlock E, Presson AP, Naliboff BD, Mayer EA, Chang L. Association between Early Adverse Life Events and Irritable Bowel Syndrome.ClinGastroenterolHepatol. 2011 Dec 15. [Epub ahead of print]

[155] Yang et al. Schisandrachinensis reverses visceral hypersensitivity in a neonatal–maternal separated rat model. J Phytomedicine November 2011.

[156] Whitehead WE. GASTROINTESTINAL MOTILITY DISORDERS OF THE SMALL INTESTINE, LARGE INTESTINE, RECTUM, AND PELVIC FLOOR. IFFGD Fact Sheet No. 162; 2001.

[157] http://www.med.unc.edu/ibs/files/educational-gi-handouts/GI%20Motility%20Functions.pdf. Accessed 22 Oct 2013.

[158] O'Malley D, Quigley EM, Dinan TG, Cryan JF. Do interactions between stress and immune responses lead to symptom exacerbations in irritable bowel syndrome? Brain Behav Immun. 2011 Oct;25(7):1333-41. Epub 2011 Apr 23.

[159] O'Malley D, Quigley EM, Dinan TG, Cryan JF. Do interactions between stress and immune responses lead to symptom exacerbations in irritable bowel syndrome? Brain Behav Immun. 2011 Oct;25(7):1333-41. Epub 2011 Apr 23.

[160] Saini R, Saini S, Sharma S. Potential of probiotics in controlling cardiovascular diseases. *J Cardiovasc Dis Res.* 2010

Oct-Dec; 1(4): 213–214.

161 http://chriskresser.com/the-high-price-of-antibiotic-use-can-our-guts-ever-fully-recover. Accessed 18 Oct 2013.

162 Schwartz S, Friedberg I, Ivanov I, Davidson LA, Goldsby JS, Dahl DB, Herman D, Wang M, Donovan SM and Chapkin R. A Metagenomic Study of Diet-Dependent Interaction Between Gut Microbiota and Host in Infants Reveals Differences in Immune Response. GENOME BIOLOGY, April 2012

163 Kronman MP, Zaoutis TE, Haynes K, Feng R, Coffin SE. Antibiotic Exposure and IBD Development Among Children: A Population-Based Cohort Study. *Pediatrics* 2012 Oct;130(4):e794-803

164 C. Codling, L. O'Mahony, F. Shanahan, E.M. Quigley, J.R. Marchesi. A molecular analysis of fecal and mucosal bacterial communities in irritable bowel syndrome. Dig. Dis. Sci., 55 (2011), pp. 392–397

165 Johannesson E, Simrén M, Strid H, Bajor A, Sadik R. Physical activity improves symptoms in irritable bowel syndrome: a randomized controlled trial. Am J Gastroenterol. 2011 May;106(5):915-22. Epub 2011 Jan 4.

166 Daley AJ, Grimmett C, Roberts L, Wilson S, Fatek M, Roalfe A, Singh S. The effects of exercise upon symptoms and quality of life in patients diagnosed with irritable bowel syndrome: a randomised controlled trial. Int J Sports Med. 2008 Sep;29(9):778-82. Epub 2008 May 6.

167 Zhou HQ, Yao M, Chen GY, Ding XD, Chen YP, Li DG. Functional gastrointestinal disorders among adolescents with poor sleep: a school-based study in Shanghai, China.Sleep Breath. 2011 Dec 22. [Epub ahead of print]

168 Bellini M, Gemignani A, Gambaccini D, Toti S, Menicucci D, Stasi C, Costa F, Mumolo MG, Ricchiuti A, Bedini R, de BortoliN, Marchi S. Evaluation of latent links between irritable bowel syndrome and sleep quality.World J Gastroenterol. 2011 Dec 14;17(46):5089-96.

169 Chen CL, Liu TT, Yi CH, Orr WC. Evidence for altered anorectal function in irritable bowel syndrome patients with sleep disturbance.Digestion. 2011;84(3):247-51. Epub 2011 Sep 22.

170 Konturek PC, Brzozowski T, Konturek SJ. Gut clock: implication of circadian rhythms in the gastrointestinal tract.JPhysiolPharmacol. 2011 Apr;62(2):139-50.

171 Konturek PC, Brzozowski T, Konturek SJ. Gut clock: implication of circadian rhythms in the gastrointestinal tract.JPhysiolPharmacol. 2011 Apr;62(2):139-50.

172 Spiller, RC. Potential future therapies for Irritable Bowel Syndrome: Will Disease Modifying Therapy as Opposed to Symptomatic Control Become a Reality? GastroenterolClin N Am 34 (2005) 337–354

173 Tarrerias AL, Costil V, Vicari F, Létard JC, Adenis-Lamarre P, Aisène A, Batistelli D, et al. The Effect of Inactivated

Lactobacillus LB Fermented Culture Medium on Symptom Severity: Observational Investigation in 297 Patients with Diarrhea-Predominant Irritable Bowel Syndrome. Dig Dis. 2011;29(6):588-91. Epub 2011 Dec 12.

[174]Spiller, RC. Potential future therapies for Irritable Bowel Syndrome: Will Disease Modifying Therapy as Opposed to Symptomatic Control Become a Reality? GastroenterolClin N Am 34 (2005) 337–354

[175] Peltonen R, Nenonen M, Helve T, Hänninen O, Toivanen P, Eerola E. Faecal microbial flora and disease activity in rheumatoid arthritis during a vegan diet. *Rheumatology* (1997) 36 (1): 64-68. doi: 10.1093/rheumatology/36.1.64

[176]Doll R, Peto R. The causes of cancer: quantitative estimates of avoidable risks of cancer in the United States today. J Natl Cancer Inst. 1981;66:1191–308

[177]O'Keefe SJD, Chung D, Mahmoud N, Sepulveda AR, Manafe M, Arch J, Adada, H, van der Merwe T. Why Do African Americans Get More Colon Cancer than Native Africans? J. Nutr. January 2007 137: 175S-182S

[178] O'Keefe SJ. Nutrition and Colonic Health: The Critical Role of the Microbiota. *Curr Opin Gastroenterol.* 2008;24(1):51-58.

[179] Koeth, R., Wang, Z., Levison, B., Buffa, J., Org, E., Sheehy, B., Britt, E., Fu, X., Wu, Y., Li, L., Smith, J., DiDonato, J., Chen, J., Li, H., Wu, G., Lewis, J., Warrier, M., Brown, J., Krauss, R., Tang, W., Bushman, F., Lusis, A., & Hazen, S. (2013). Intestinal microbiota metabolism of l-carnitine, a nutrient in red meat, promotes atherosclerosis Nature Medicine DOI: 10.1038/nm.3145

[180]Ruepert L, Quartero AO, de Wit NJ, van der Heijden GJ, Rubin G, Muris JW. Bulking agents, antispasmodics and antidepressants for the treatment of irritable bowel syndrome. Cochrane Database Syst Rev. 2011 Aug 10;(8):CD003460.

[181] Kaminski A, Kamper A, Thaler K, Chapman A, Gartlehner G. Antidepressants for the treatment of abdominal pain-related functional gastrointestinal disorders in children and adolescents. Cochrane Database Syst Rev. 2011 Jul 6;(7):CD008013.

[182]Tarrerias AL, Costil V, Vicari F, Létard JC, Adenis-Lamarre P, Aisène A, Batistelli D, et al. The Effect of Inactivated Lactobacillus LB Fermented Culture Medium on Symptom Severity: Observational Investigation in 297 Patients with Diarrhea-Predominant Irritable Bowel Syndrome. Dig Dis. 2011;29(6):588-91. Epub 2011 Dec 12.

[183] Horvath A, Dziechciarz P, Szajewska H. Meta-analysis: Lactobacillus rhamnosus GG for abdominal pain-related functional gastrointestinal disorders in childhood. Aliment PharmacolTher. 2011 Jun;33(12):1302-10. doi: 10.1111/j.1365-2036.2011.04665.x. Epub 2011 Apr 20.

184Spiller, RC. Potential future therapies for Irritable Bowel Syndrome: Will Disease Modifying Therapy as Opposed to Symptomatic Control Become a Reality? GastroenterolClin N Am 34 (2005) 337–354

185Bortolotti M, Porta S. Effect of red pepper on symptoms of irritable bowel syndrome: preliminary study. Dig Dis Sci. 2011 Nov;56(11):3288-95. Epub 2011 May 15.

186Walker AF, Middleton RW, Petrowicz O. Artichoke leaf extract reduces symptoms of irritable bowel syndrome in a post-marketing surveillance study. Phytother Res. 2001 Feb;15(1):58-61.

187 McKay DL, Blumberg JB. A review of the bioactivity and potential health benefits of peppermint tea (Menthapiperita L.). Phytother Res. 2006 Aug;20(8):619-33.

188 Monk JM, Kim W, Callaway E, Turk HF, Foreman JE, Peters JM, He W, Weeks B, Alaniz RC, McMurray DN, Chapkin RS. Immunomodulatory action of dietary fish oil and targeted deletion of intestinal epithelial cell PPARδ in inflammation-induced colon carcinogenesis. Am J PhysiolGastrointest Liver Physiol. 2012 Jan;302(1):G153-67. Epub 2011 Sep 22.

189 Zhou Q, Souba WW, Croce CM, Verne GN. MicroRNA-29a regulates intestinal membrane permeability in patients with irritable bowel syndrome. Gut. 2010 Jun;59(6):775-84. Epub 2009 Dec 1.

190 Johnson PM, Kenny PJ. *Nat Neurosci.* 2010;13:635–641.

191 Newman L, Haryono R, Keast R. Functionality of fatty acid chemoreception: a potential factor in the development of obesity? *Nutrients.* 2013 Apr 17;5(4):1287-300.

cxcii Sharot et al. Dopamine Enhances Expectation of Pleasure in Humans. *Current Biology*, 2009; DOI: 10.1016/j.cub.2009.10.025

cxciii Strack F, Martin LL, Stepper S. Inhibiting and facilitating conditions of the human smile: a nonobtrusive test of the facial feedback hypothesis. *J Pers Soc Psychol.* 1988 May;54(5):768-77.